AND A
BANG
ON THE
EAR

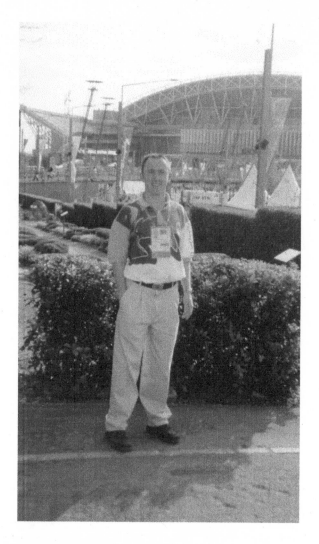

PHIL QUINLAN played every sport shown on TV and represented his county in cross-country twice, but his life was suddenly and irreparably changed by a clash of heads playing football. Having defied the twenty-five percent odds of surviving, living with a disability, travelling the globe, finding love, Phil hopes his story is an inspirational one. Through all the hurt, rage and rehabilitation, trials and tribulations, he's living the dream now …

STEVE O'ROURKE is a writer and former journalist. With bylines in *Hot Press*, The42 and ESPN, he has interviewed musicians, politicians and Olympians. Once Ireland's only full-time NFL journalist, he has always believed that sport produces the best human-interest stories and has dedicated his career to bringing those stories to life. He currently lives in Dublin with his wife and two children, and works in advertising.

AND A
PHIL QUINLAN WITH STEVE O'ROURKE
BANG
RECLAIMING MY LIFE AFTER A BRAIN INJURY
ON THE
FOREWORD BY PAUL HOWARD
EAR

THE O'BRIEN PRESS
DUBLIN

First published 2023 by The O'Brien Press Ltd,
12 Terenure Road East, Rathgar, Dublin 6, D06 HD27, Ireland.
Tel: +353 1 4923333; Fax: +353 1 4922777
E-mail: books@obrien.ie. Website: obrien.ie
The O'Brien Press is a member of Publishing Ireland.

ISBN: 978-1-78849-322-2

Text © Phil Quinlan 2023
The moral rights of the author have been asserted.
Editing, typesetting, layout, design © The O'Brien Press Ltd

Cover and inside design by Emma Byrne.

8 7 6 5 4 3 2 1
27 26 25 24 23

Printed and bound by Scandbook AB, Sweden.
The paper in this book is produced using pulp from managed forests.

Published in

DUBLIN
UNESCO
City of Literature

Great Irish books
O'BRIEN
obrien.ie

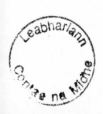

Dedication

For Mam and Dad, who dragged me through the first half ...

For Helena, Eileen and Joe, who are hauling me through the second half and injury time ...

CONTENTS

FOREWORD

This could have been an altogether different book. Were it not for the cruellest of accidents, you could have in your hands the autobiography of Phil Quinlan, Premier League footballer, Olympic gold medal-winning triathlete or record Irish try-scorer. Instead, it's a book about how a young boy's dreams were sundered by rotten luck and how his adult self battled and eventually succeeded in reaching an accommodation with that.

Most of us who love sport grew up playing out scenarios in our minds that placed us centre stage in some heroic drama or other. We imagined ourselves scoring the winning goal in a World Cup final, breasting the line first at the end of a 100-metre sprint, or throwing a right hook out of nowhere to put the world heavyweight champion on the seat of his pants.

For most of us, our dreams remained just that. In my case, poor eyesight and puniness, as well as physical and moral cowardice, put paid to my sporting ambitions, such as they ever were. By the time I was fourteen, I knew that if I was going to be involved in sport, it would be as an observer, although if I worked really hard, I thought, I might persuade a newspaper to pay me to observe it.

No child grows up dreaming of sitting on a side-line with a laptop computer, of course, but that was the adjustment I had to make because of the various ways in which nature short-changed me. I am fifty-two years of age and I am just about okay with it now.

Some dreams break on bigger rocks. Like Phil Quinlan's. On a foggy day in 1989, while playing for Parkvilla against Torro United, he rose to head a ball and sustained an injury that sounded as innocuous as it's described in the title of this book. We've all knocked heads with someone else. Usually, you stand up, feeling dazed and sore, and you carry on. But sometimes it doesn't happen like that. Phil's was one of those freak injuries that couldn't be 'run off'.

It left him in a coma with a one-in-four chance of survival. He beat the odds but woke from his sinister sleep to discover that his challenges were no longer evading tackles, or jumping hurdles, or beating a centre-half for pace. They were more mundane goals, like learning to walk again – 'barefoot on broken glass' is the phrase he uses to describe the experience – and learning to live with the knowledge of what was lost while he set about – in another memorable phrase – 'wobbling around the world'.

The story contained within these covers isn't the conventional tale of sporting triumph. There is no *Rocky II* ending. It's about a different kind of triumph, less dramatic perhaps, less televisual certainly, but no less heroic. It's a story of adaptation and in the end acceptance.

In these pages, we watch the process unfold as if in real time. The journey takes us to some extraordinary places, through the voluntary work, travels and relationships that added perspective to his experience. We also meet the entire *dramatis personae* of his story, including the medical staff who attended to him and the boy – now man – whose head delivered the accidental bang on the ear that left him with a lifetime of pain and paralysis.

There is rage and bitterness and self-pity in these pages. But what would a story like this be worth without those elements? He deals with the legacy of what happened to him in a way that is both real and deeply moving. In one especially harrowing piece, he talks of 'sitting here pretending I'm okay, when all I can think is, "What doesn't kill you sometimes makes you wish it had."'

We get nothing less than the full gamut of emotions that he went through. There are moments in this book that made me feel uplifted and others that broke my heart like a coconut. Tempering his anger is his gradual discovery of the scattergun cruelty of life, as people he loved – and considered fortunate not to have an affliction like his – had their own lives snuffed out just as suddenly and as senselessly as his was catastrophically altered.

And through all the pages of painful self-examination and self-discovery, his passion for sport remains undimmed. So many of his memories are defined and coloured by his love of football, rugby, Gaelic and athletics. He recalls reading Paul McGrath's autobiography on the day he lost his virginity. He remembers a painful relationship break-up that happened after a cinema date to see, of all movies, *Jerry Maguire*. Sporting events are his ordinances. The points on his compass.

In his dreams, Phil still runs the length of Kalungwishi Street in the Zambia of his childhood, hunting down John Ngugi and Dieter Baumann to win gold for Ireland, even as the morning brings the inevitable, waking realisation that he's a disabled, middle-aged man now. But there's also the consolation of watching his children fall headlong in love with sport just as he did at their age.

This is an extraordinary memoir of a sporting life curtailed. It doesn't end with a Grand Slam, or an Olympic medal, or a winning goal in an All Ireland football final. But those of us who love sport know that most of its greatest heroes have never stood on a victory rostrum.

This is the story of Phil Quinlan. It's unlikely you've ever heard of him before. But by the time you finish this book, you won't forget him.

Paul Howard, January 2023

EVERY STEP YOU TAKE

Mam and Dad are nervously watching me attempt my first steps. I don't know how I know, but I know. I suppose they're nervous because they're that little bit older now, older than most to be wondering what the following weeks, months, and years have in store if I can just put one foot in front of the other. That's going to be easier said than done, of course. My brain is firing signal after signal, but it's not quite working the way it should and the signals are getting lost on the way to my feet.

Still, in the back of my mind I want Mam and Dad to be proud. I want them to know that if I can do this, I can do anything. I think about my dog at home, Lucky, and how I might get to play with him if I can just get from this side of the room to the other. It's only five metres but, right now, it might as well be five miles.

It's sometimes hard to believe the moment ever happened; that I was ever in the middle of all that love, and belief, and possibility, because now I'm not. The love was real, I know that because I can still feel it thirty years later. The belief, however, was a disguise; some kid in a black bin bag and plastic mask worn to stop myself realising I was living in blind hope, not expectation. And as for possibility, well, anyone who tells you possibilities are endless has never spent their life waiting for Meath to lift the Liam MacCarthy Cup.

I catch Dad's eye; he's trying his best not to show it, but he's apprehensive. I know the look. It was the same one he wore when Ireland travelled to Valletta to take on Malta a few months ago. Win, and Ireland would be off to their first World Cup. Lose, and Jack Charlton would have lots of questions to answer with names like Ray Houghton, Paul McGrath and Tony Cascarino in the team. And yet the man to send my dad, and the country, into raptures that day was John Aldridge – a player who'd only found the net once in twenty-eight games for Ireland. For me, I don't just want to watch the World Cup; I want to play in it. But I won't be finding the back of the net any time soon. In fact, right now I'd settle for finding my footing.

Mam wears her emotions more openly, drifting between love and fear, excitement and worry. She's done everything in her power to get these legs of mine working. Spending ages telling me I'd be walking soon; rubbing my legs to get the feeling into my feet. Scribbling into that diary of hers or going to mass after mass after mass; the only things she's spent more money on than scratch cards are candles.

'We'll get there,' she told herself as much as me. Even more than Dad, she saw my progress – and regression – every day. She was there when I returned from the operation, in a coma. She was there when I had my first ice cream, having not eaten anything in two months. Yesterday, she was there as I managed, with a lot of help, to get out of the chair three times. I'd even put one foot on the ground.

She'd also told me that if I sorted the walking I could get my hair cut any way I wanted. I'd spotted Vinnie Jones in a football annual, Match or something like it. He was with Leeds at the time and had his head shaved at the side, with this mop of hair on the top. You see the same haircut on every Sunday League footballer and Nicky Rackard hurler today, but in 1990 it was unique.

But even the promise of a new hairdo wasn't enough to get my feet to listen to my brain in time to walk unaided for my sixteenth birthday. The date wasn't important of course, and yet it meant everything. Ever since I'd regained consciousness, some six weeks after I woke from a coma, I knew I needed to learn to walk unaided again. That day, I set a goal to do so by my sixteenth birthday. But 7 February came and went and I still wasn't walking. I did get a pair of runners – ironically enough, from Colm O'Rourke, I suppose – two tracksuits, and a Commodore 64. And I had visitors from Edenderry, Navan and Dublin that day. I even received cards from all the nurses and doctors in the hospital, though I suspect some of them were bribes to get me to give them a go on my computer.

There was one present I didn't look for, but had to open anyway: pain. The pain is there when I'm lying down. The pain is there when they are washing me in my hospital bed. The pain is there when I'm just thinking about walking, so you can imagine what the pain is like today when I'm actually trying to walk.

But I'm determined to take my first steps because in my dreams I can still run, my legs still work the way they were supposed to and so I'm flying about this way and that. But dreams are just lies we tell ourselves to help us sleep. The reality is that I'm in Beaumont Hospital, three months removed from the injury that changed my life. An accident that I know occurred but can't quite piece together.

Right now though, I want to move on from the injury. I want to walk. I have to walk.

If I can show everyone that I can start walking by myself again, they'll let me move to the National Rehabilitation Centre in Dún Laoghaire. The rehabilitation there is all based around sport. It will be perfect for me.

If I can show everyone that I can start walking by myself again, they'll let me play rugby. There's a spot in the starting XV at Lansdowne Road up for grabs. It will be perfect for me.

If I can show everyone that I can start walking by myself again, this whole thing will be chalked up as just a bang on the ear. There's a whole world of possibilities out there if I can get my foot to hit the floor. It will be perfect for me.

I look my parents in the eyes. I nod. And I lift my left leg ...

CHAPTER 1

SOME THINGS HURT MORE, MUCH MORE, THAN CARS AND GIRLS

26 NOVEMBER 1989 – TWENTY-FOUR MINUTES AFTER THE INJURY

We'd gone a goal up, Bundles (Roy Newman) was the scorer. 'Do something, Neville,' our coach Gerry Brown was roaring at Neville Dunne. Not great instructions, but pretty indicative of the general apathy all of us were feeling about playing on a damp, miserable November afternoon.

That's when I noticed Philip. As disinterested as Neville was, Philip was wandering around the pitch aimlessly. I knew he'd taken a knock earlier in the game, but he seemed to shake it off right enough. 'Jesus, will you cop yourself on, Philip,' I said to myself. It was bad enough Gerry was going to give us a bollocking for Neville's performance, I didn't need him gathering any more ammunition.

Gerry had noticed though, and hauled Philip off at half-time. About five minutes into the second half, one of the lads noticed that Philip had fallen asleep in the dugout. We all started laughing and making fun of him. He was in for it now, once Gerry spotted him.

Within seconds though, the mood shifted dramatically. Someone tried to wake Philip, but he wouldn't stir. There was blood coming from his ear. 'He's dead,' someone said. 'Philip is dead.'

John Brady, Parkvilla teammate

AUTUMN 1977 – ELEVEN YEARS BEFORE THE INJURY

Mine was a typical childhood. Born in Limerick. Moved to Navan. Started school in Zambia. Maybe not all that typical actually, but it goes some way towards explaining how a child can be lining out in his imagination for Munster against the All Blacks one minute, and beating the great Kenyans over 5,000 metres the next.

We ended up in Zambia – 151 Kalungwishi Street, Kitwe, to be exact – because Dad had been told an opportunity had come up, but it would mean moving his young family. Zambia had relied on mining for its economic development ever since commercial mining began in 1928, and copper mines are still a major source of revenue for the country. But the 1960s and 1970s were decades of high metal demand, high mineral prices, high production and high rewards. Dad couldn't really turn it down. Zambia was where the action was.

Not that I was complaining, because I loved every minute of it. We had a huge front garden – which felt to me like it had room for Thomond Park and a bit to spare – with a massive gate leading into it. The back garden was roughly the same size, but its most striking feature was a mango tree made for climbing right in the middle, while the end of the garden was fenced off by banana trees and sugar canes.

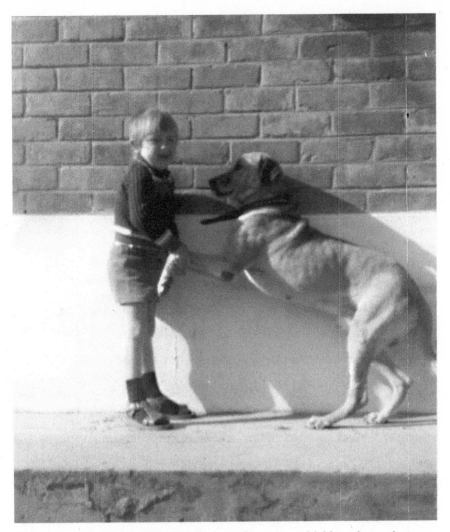

My love of dogs started in Zambia as a four-year-old. Here I am playing with Becky, our Rhodesian Ridgeback.

I was obsessed with climbing at that age. The mango tree could become a cliff face. The front gate could become a mountain. Mount Mumpu could become Everest. At first, just climbing the tree was enough. But then I'd look for a slightly more difficult route, just to challenge myself. By the time we left, it's a wonder I wasn't trying to climb the thing with just my feet.

While life in Zambia was all about playing outside, it wasn't without its risks. My friend Anthony had a pal who owned a mini-motorbike. One day, we all thought it would be a great idea to tie a rope from that motorbike to my bicycle. It started brilliantly, as off he sped with me in tow clinging to the handlebars, my exhilaration in tune with his acceleration. It was only when we were approaching the first corner that I spotted the fatal flaw in our plan. If he stopped, there was no way for me to stop in time. Terrified, I figured the only way to escape was to fling myself off my bicycle, landing head first in the ditch. I tore my face asunder and the bruises on my body resembled a map of one of Dad's mines.

When I got home, Mam and Dad were getting ready for a night out, probably at Diggers Rugby Club, and wanted to cancel because I looked so battered and broken. I told them to go, but one of the cuts I gave myself obviously became infected because that night I needed a fan to calm my temperature. I eventually made a full recovery, but my Evel Knievel days were done.

Instead, I stuck to the climbing, fueling my expeditions with Fanta and salty biltong. None of the fancy hipster stuff you get now either, but a 12-inch piece of sun dried beef that looked like a wooden ruler and some people said tasted just as good. I loved it though, even if it took hours to eat. Sometimes, when my mind wanders, I'm still a climber.

Kitwe came into existence in 1936, an insignificant stop on the railway Cecil Rhodes was building to support the British Empire's expanding copper mining interests in Africa. However, as the copper industry grew, so did Kitwe and by the time my family arrived there in 1977, it was a bustling city in a country that was then called Rhodesia. And while most of Rhodesia became Zimbabwe, Kitwe has been part of Zambia since 1964.

Sport was huge in Kitwe. There was a cricket ground that had famously played host to two first-class matches in the sixties, the only first-class cricket ever played in Zambia. There were no fewer than three big football teams; Power Dynamos FC, Nkana FC, and Kitwe United. Both union and league rugby was played, albeit at a lower level and most of the adults seemed more interested in the post game entertainment than the sport itself.

But for me, when I wasn't running, I was swimming. And while lots of people preferred the bigger Nkana Mine Pool in the centre of the city, the smaller pool at the Italian Club was much more my style.

I had taught myself to swim earlier that year, not by swimming side to side like everyone told me to, but by swimming lengths, and grabbing onto the side whenever I needed to come up for air. Eventually the number of times I had to surface was reduced to zero and, within a few weeks, I was swimming back-to-back lengths of the pool.

Of course, being a naturally competitive child, that wasn't enough to keep me happy for very long so I started to challenge myself by seeing how long I could stay under the water without breathing. The easiest way I found to do this was not by counting seconds, but instead seeing how many coins I could pick up from the bottom of the pool without pausing to take a breath.

One particular day Keith, whose family lived directly opposite our house on Kalungwishi Street, and his Mam decided to join us at the Italian Club. Because of their proximity, Keith's family and mine would often spend time in each other's company. Sometimes that involved reminiscing about home, but often it was just two Irish families discussing the unique circumstances they found themselves in.

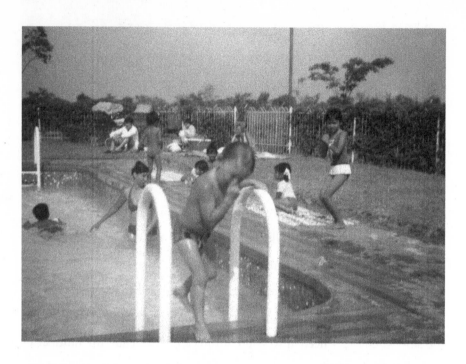

Above: Getting out of the pool after another famous dive in Zambia.
Below: The Rokana mine swimming pool when I revisited in 2004.

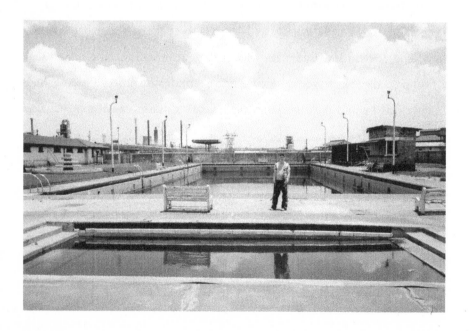

While I was scrawny and long, the proverbial butcher's pencil, Keith was broad and hard as nails. I explained to him the challenge of collecting the coins from the bottom of the pool, and wondered aloud if he was really built to beat my record in a bid to ensure he'd challenge me. I was only delighted with myself when he decided he'd collect way more coins than I could.

After I'd taken my turn and set a new personal best, I climbed out of the pool. But when I turned around, I noticed that Keith was calling his mam who – deep in conversation with my own – failed to see or hear her son's pleas for help.

'Look Mam, Keith can't swim,' I shouted as I dove back in to the pool. He was about 10m away from me, but I took a deep breath and breast-stroked my way underwater to grab his arm. He struggled a bit at first, but once I had a firm grip I pulled him to the surface with all my might.

At this stage, both our mothers had noticed the commotion and were frantic by the poolside. Keith's Mam pulled him out of the water and, once she'd established he was okay, unleashed an unmighty smack across his arse. Her reaction was out of pure fear, of course, but I couldn't help but think Keith would rather still be in the water.

And the hero of the hour? Well I was handed a bottle of Fanta and told to be more careful going after those coins. Lying in bed that night, I considered mortality for the first time. What if Keith had died? How could anyone ever recover from their friend dying?

CHAPTER 2

RUNNING UP THAT HILL

26 NOVEMBER 1989 – TWO HOURS AFTER THE INJURY

We were in Trim, in the pub, and I got the phone call to say, 'Philip is in hospital after the match.'

I said to Angela: 'How bad can it be; he probably just broke his leg.' I'd never seen anyone take a bang on the ear playing football. Even in rugby, the only time I'd ever seen anything like it was when Jimmy Orr landed on the point of the ball in Diggers.

When we were driving to Beaumont, we were shitting it. There's no other way to describe it. Angela was there holding an unlit cigarette in her hand the whole way. She couldn't get the lighter to work.

Then seeing Philip lying there in the hospital. It was savage. I was just in bits. We didn't know if you were going to make it. The priest was around. There were people praying for him in the church. There were even people who thought Philip was already gone. That was hard.

When he got home from the hospital, the biggest impact was on James, his brother. James would have been big into the football too and now that Philip wasn't able to play with him he was just a bit confused by it all.

But it had an effect on us all. People may have thought that I could go to work to kind of escape having to think about it, but it didn't mean I did. But Angela and the girls, they were the ones home with Philip all the time, so I suppose it had a bigger impact on them.

The thing is, before the injury, we were going okay. I was making a few bob. The kids were all well. We were happy. It goes to show you that everything, everything, can change in an instant.

Once in a blue moon, I do wonder to myself, 'What if?' Philip would have been a player. He was a brilliant athlete. But you let those thoughts go quickly; there's no point letting them sit there to fester.

Jim Quinlan, father of Phil

SPRING 1998 – NINE YEARS AFTER THE INJURY

I'm preparing for my latest expedition out from number 57 Mountjoy Square – a 140-metre walk to the Hill 16 pub in order to catch 'Match of the Day'. My housemate thinks I'm mad. The heavens have opened outside. 'You'll catch your death,' he says. He just can't understand how I can still love football the way I do, after everything it took away from me nine years ago.

I call it an expedition, though for most people, it's a few minutes' stroll. For me, now, it takes planning, endurance and all the concentration I can muster. Despite the tempest, I can't resist my temptress, so I slip on my shoes and I start to wobble my way down to Gardiner Street. I don't mind spending money on good shoes. These ones are brown, ECCO I think. Because of the way I walk – pushing off my right toes – that shoe always wears a little quicker than the left. These ones still have a few months left in them though.

Even with the wind and the rain, I'm only a few steps down the road before I'm sweating. Sweating a lot more than I should. The concentration required is immense because of my equinus – a condition that makes me walk on my toes and keeps me off balance. For each step, I have to think about lifting my right leg. Next, I have to think about keeping that leg in the air without it spasming and launching off towards the canal. Finally, I have to think about how and where I'm going to place my leg back on the ground. I have to do this for every step.

I'm about forty-three steps in – you learn to count when they're so energy consuming – when my leg suddenly freezes for no good reason. It must know I'm running late if I want to make it to the pub in time for the highlights of the first game. When it freezes like this, I can't react quickly enough to stabilise myself. My body tenses, ready for the inevitable. All I can do most of the time is hope I hit the grass, but I'm often just as likely to land on the path or the road. Thankfully, after only a speed wobble, it comes back under control. With a lot of effort, I place it carefully on the ground and get ready for step number forty-four.

Despite the weather, the rest of the walk is uneventful until I make it to just across the road from the pub. But, like a climber attempting to scale Everest, I need to be extra careful here. Summit fever is real, but I'm in the Death Zone now and I have the Second Step to negotiate. While Gardiner Street's skyline doesn't feature Kanchenjunga, Lhotse or Makalu, it's just as dangerous, because now I have to try and cross the road safely.

I'm also not lucky enough to have had a team of Nepalese climbers install a ladder for me to reduce the difficulty. Instead, everything that could be against me, is. The incline of the slope has my right leg trembling. The rain has turned the smooth tarmac into an ice sheet. And there's a wind blowing down towards the Liffey that feels like it might take me with it. I breathe in deeply, holding my breath, and I think about stepping down off the path.

Fifteen seconds later, I exhale, and my body responds to my brain's commands after completing the advanced calculus required to make the four-inch drop. I wonder once again how differently people might treat me if they could read my mind at moments like this, as I decide which foot is better to land with, or ask myself if I'll do more harm than good by holding onto the bonnet of a parked car. Tonight, the big question is whether I should wait until the wind dies down.

Questions. Doubts. Fears.

All of which means that every decision is slow and deliberate. And even then my nerves don't always hold. Sometimes my body is kidnapped by my spasticity and, if I can't pay the ransom in time, leaves me on my arse on the ground. As if that's not enough, I then have to spend ten very awkward seconds trying to find my way back to my feet, apologising for my existence.

There's no sign of the wind dying down. I'm just going to have to go for it. 'Don't freak out,' I tell myself as I place my left foot on the road, swinging my right around after it. Success. This time it has planted firmly on the tarmac and seems to be behaving itself. I wait two seconds though, just to be sure.

One.

Two.

I've made it, but as always, success is short lived. There's still the matter of crossing the road. A car has slowed down to my right, letting me cross. I stop to give the driver a thumbs up. I don't look at the car face on. Normally I make certain to thank drivers for slowing down, for understanding that I need extra time to make my way across the road. But I'm exhausted now.

And turning my head means potentially losing my balance. I'm so close now I can't risk it. So, on I stride, slowly, carefully. Totally focused on landing one safe step after another. 'Don't fall,' I say quietly to myself. Inside, I scream the same words.

By the time I reach the far side of the road, I'm drenched in sweat as much as rain. I pause momentarily. Stepping up onto a kerb is easier than stepping down, but it still brings its risks. I plant my left leg first as an anchor, leaving my spastic leg behind me and hoping it behaves. It does, thankfully, and a few minutes later I reach the door of the pub.

I'm delighted with myself. Most Irish people dream of climbing the steps of the Hogan Stand to lift Sam or Liam, but I'm celebrating making it to the Hill 16 pub. My coat, the love child of a dalliance between Jack Charlton's and John Motson's, is soaked as I take it off and take in the floor plan ahead of me. I still need to actually make it to the bar after all. Thankfully, the wooden floor looks like it hasn't seen a polish since John Paul II told us he loved us all, so that should make it easier to traverse. The smell of stale cigarette smoke hangs in the air as I use free chairs to make my way up to the bar. There's barely anyone else here, so that makes it a little easier.

The television in the corner is already playing 'Match of the Day'. By my watch, I reckon I've missed the day's big game, but there's still plenty of action to catch. I'm not a big drinker – it doesn't pay to be when every step in these conditions is a lottery, so I order a rock shandy. My voice, at least since 1989, has always been more of a whisper than a hurricane and I'm not sure the barman has heard me. I haul myself up into my seat, getting comfortable for the football, and ask him again.

He scowls.

'I think you've had enough,' he says.

I look around, flabbergasted. He *must* be serving someone else behind me. But there's nobody else he could be talking to.

On the television, the crowd erupts. Somebody has scored, but I've no idea who. All I can see now is the barman, staring right at me, thinking I'm drunk.

'I saw you stumbling in,' he says. 'You've had enough.'

I continue to look at him in silent disbelief. He's now pointing, first at my coat, then at the door. He thinks I'm pissed. I go to speak, but he cuts me off. 'I said,' his voice rising, 'I think you've had enough. Please get out.'

The back of my eyes are burning. All I wanted was a quiet rock shandy and to watch the football, and here is some fucker accusing me of being drunk when I'm sober enough to take confession. To make matters worse, his eyes are full of confrontation, and something more than that. There's a look in them that screams out that he thinks he's better than me. That here is just another drunk, wasting his life. But he doesn't know the first thing about me. He doesn't know me from Adam. I hate confrontation, but I'm tired of this. Something snaps.

'I'm disabled,' I say with all the force I can muster.

'What?'

'I said, I'm disabled. I'm not drunk.'

I can hear his brain working. Putting together the last few minutes like a toddler with a Rubik's Cube; from the moment I wobbled into the bar to the time I ordered my drink. Something in him changes, slowly, as it dawns on him that I am telling the truth.

'Match of the Day' continues, with the Liverpool game up next, and his cheeks now match their jerseys. But he doesn't say sorry. He doesn't say anything at all. Instead he pours my rock shandy, places it silently in front of me, and takes the £5 note out of my hand. He drops the change back in front of me with a level of self-righteousness that only those who know they are wholly wrong can achieve.

I stay for the full length of 'Match of the Day', but he doesn't come near me again, doesn't ask me if I want another drink. I'd like to tell you I stayed to prove a point, to show him that you shouldn't judge a book by its cover or a man by his wobble.

But the truth is I don't know what else I can do. If I leave in a huff, he's won. If I give him a piece of my mind he can kick me out for causing trouble. And besides, I'm bolloxed from the walk down and I don't fancy turning around straight away to trek home.

Deep down I know he should apologise to me, but I don't have the words yet to ask for that apology. Maybe I never will? Instead, I sit silently through the football, slowly sipping on my one rock shandy, and he and I steal glimpses at one another until Des Lynam blows the final whistle.

The walk home is a little easier, despite conditions worsening. It's always been less difficult for me to contend with an uphill walk; the risk of falling is not as bad when you know you're almost guaranteed to go forward. But with every step, the barman's words ring in my ear.

'I saw you stumbling in.' Step.

'You've had enough.' Step.

'Please get out.' Step.

By the time I reached the green door of number 57, I can barely contain my rage. My housemate says something to me but I've headed straight to my room. When I close the door the floodgates open. Does everyone think about me this way? Is this why people won't approach me, because they think I'm drunk?

That fucking bastard. How fucking dare he. My tears have emptied, but my heart is still full of rage, I lash out. I start punching myself, screaming at myself for being a worthless cripple who doesn't deserve to be treated fairly.

But I didn't choose this. I didn't ask for any of this.

I just wanted to go and watch a football match. Nine years ago, all I wanted to do was to go play a football match. And that's when everything changed. Changed completely.

CHAPTER 3

GIVE HIM A BALL (AND A YARD OF GRASS)

27 NOVEMBER 1989 – TWENTY-FOUR HOURS AFTER THE INJURY

Jim left him to Round O at 1.15pm. Football at 2pm. Got hurt (clash of heads) at 2:35pm.

Arrived at Navan Hospital at 4pm. Later arrived at Beaumont. Had scan/operation at 7–8:30pm.

We went to see him in the ward. Left around 10pm. We stayed in Robby's. Could not sleep waiting for the phone to ring all night.

Dr Young said the operation had gone very well. Removed the clot. It was very big and there might be swelling. He gave Philip a twenty-five percent chance of living.

We were allowed in to see him after the operation. He was on all the machines and drips. His head was bandaged up. We stayed for five minutes.

Robby, Liz, Dave were in.

Philip is in a coma.

Diary of Angela Quinlan, mother of Philip Quinlan

WINTER 1981 – EIGHT YEARS BEFORE THE INJURY

Our departure from Zambia took me a little bit by surprise. I was doing really well in school, finding my feet, and flippers, as a both runner and swimmer. I'd also just made friends with Ivan Moran, an only child who lived close by and seemed to have every toy under the sun. We somehow always ended up playing at his house.

But when people talk about a person having a twinkle in their eye, they're describing Ivan. He was always up for divilment. One evening, as Mam and Dad were celebrating a win in the rugby, Ivan and myself were wandering around the car park of Diggers RFC trying to amuse ourselves. He spotted a brand new Land Rover and we decided that it would be a great idea to put stones in the petrol tank. Oh how we laughed until we realised our crime of the century had been spotted by some locals who promptly told Dad exactly what we'd been up to. Ivan put some of his mischievous nature to good use afterwards, and he's a famous special effects guy in Hollywood these days, working on some well-known movies.

Mam and Dad have never admitted that's why we ended up back in Navan, but I've often teased them that it had to play a role.

When we landed back in Silverlawns in October 1981, Nanny had already booked me into the newest school in the town, St Paul's. On my first day, I was introduced by the teacher as the young lad who used to rob bread and milk from his doorstep to make mud pies with them. As first impressions go, it was pretty memorable.

I wasn't sure I would settle in after Zambia, but I quickly came to love St Paul's and the freedom of running around playing at breaktime. Ever the competitor, I'd always tried to be first in my line, and the rivalry between myself and James Raleigh for that honour continued into secondary school.

School sports days were electric, the highlight of the year. In sixth class I finished joint first alongside Adrian Lee in the 100m sprint after a photo finish that must have been taken with a polaroid. At the medal ceremony, the school handed Adrian the gold medal, and me the silver, with the agreement that we would swap in six months. To this day I'm still waiting for the gold to be handed over.

Ever the sporting family, Dad – still fit as a fiddle from playing rugby under the blistering African sun – won the fathers' race, while Mam's softball exploits in Zambia helped her place in the mammies' version.

There was an incredible easiness to my childhood at this stage. Just like Zambia, everything was based outside, even if it was a little cooler and significantly wetter. Running, cycling, playing 'kick the can', wandering all over the estate and into the field across the road from us. Summers spent

Silverlawn Sharks, the first football team I ever joined. Maybe I should have stayed playing in goal! Photo by Joe Rice.

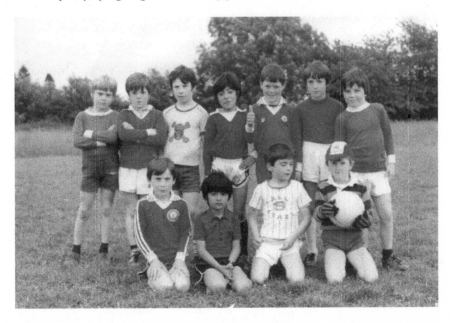

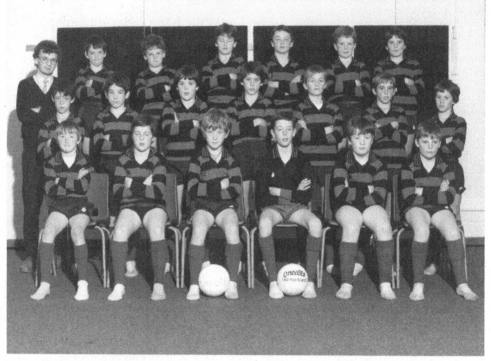

A winning St Paul's team.

making camps in the hay bales or organising my own Olympic Games just to test myself against everyone. I was fast, but never the fastest. I could go forever though and eventually joined Sean Cooney at Navan Shamrocks where I really learned how to run.

We played everything we watched; football, rugby, American football, basketball, cricket, tennis. Navan could become the San Siro, Giants Stadium or Lords, depending how we chalked the roads outside our house. Our skills may have had their limits, but our imaginations certainly didn't.

It was sports twenty-four hours a day, seven days a week, 365 days a year. Even a trip to the shops could turn into a competitive event. Colm O'Rourke had a sports shop in Navan Shopping Centre, and there was a terrific little maze close by. At our best, some of us were able to spring out of the middle of the maze in five seconds or less. Little did I know that, years later, I'd still be doing laps of the centre, but this time with the aid of a trolley.

But the winter of 1982 put a halt to everything. I was eight years old and it was my first time seeing snow. Did this happen every year? It was only when the pipes froze and we couldn't play sports that I began to grow sick of it. Turns out it would come to be known as The Big Snow, so I wouldn't have to get too used to it.

Over the next few years, I settled into life in Navan and my athletic prowess grew. I was on the Meath team for both the U12 and U14 Leinster Cross-Country Championships. I built a bit of a mystique around myself. After all, surely the boy from the same continent as the great Kenyan

Heading a ball out in the back garden as a twelve-year-old.

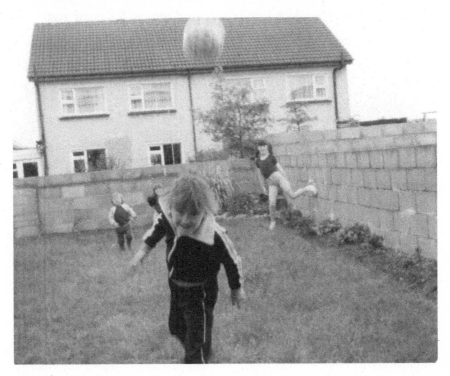

middle distance runners possessed similar abilities. The other boys didn't know I was born in Limerick.

But I could walk the walk too. At the age of fourteen, I could cover 3.2 kilometres in 13.26. I knew the exact distance because there was a turn out the Windtown Road with a gate leading to Spike Island on the river Blackwater that was exactly this distance from my house. Armed with a stopwatch, I'd either run by myself or have a mate cycle alongside me to time the run.

By fourteen, I could cover 1005 metres in 3.47 seconds, and my best time from the ESB power station out to the foodstore in Windtown and back into the house (2100 metres) was 8.25. It was just a shame that neither was an Olympic distance.

In the grey tracksuit (I always hated the cold), about to run in the Trials for the Meath team – which I made that year and the following year.

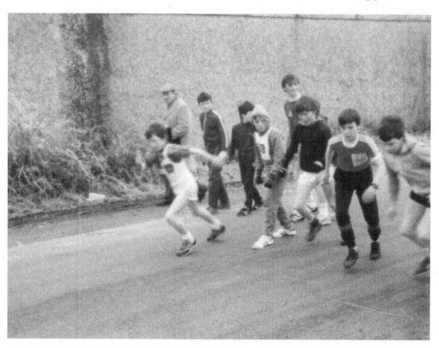

But running was more than just a way for me to exercise my competitiveness or demonstrate my prowess as an athlete. Running made me feel alive. I knew then I was always going to be a runner.

LONDON, 1987 – TWO YEARS BEFORE THE INJURY

In primary school we were given the chance to go to London. It was a reward for getting rid of all the stones buried in the muck on the front football pitch – no health-and-safety back then. The big smoke. Dublin on steroids. You can imagine the chaos as Sixth Class from St Paul's piled onto the bus in Navan. By the time we made our way to the ferry, the younger teachers were probably sorry they had volunteered. And by the time we arrived in Euston Station via Holyhead, they were probably regretting their choice of career.

Our accommodation was on the budget end of the scale, a dingy guesthouse in Kensington. The girls were staying on the floor above us in the guesthouse. We could only chat to them by risking death hanging out a window.

Of the things I'd remembered to pack, Weetabix was the most important. It had been my religious breakfast since we'd arrived home from Zambia. My record was thirteen in one sitting, but without a full supply in my trusty yellow Tupperware bowl, I didn't have much hope of beating that in London.

I asked the guesthouse owners if I could have a bowl on the first morning and, because I was quite a small kid, the manager in the guest house reached up and took out a dusty bowl from a manky cupboard. He wiped the dust with his hand and handed it to me. I looked at him in disbelief and said no thanks. It would be toast for me for a few days.

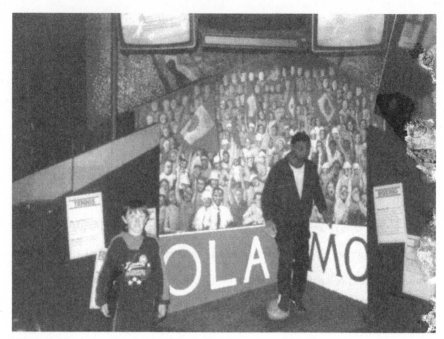

With Pelé at the Guinness World Records Museum in London on our school tour in 1987.

We took in all the usual sights. Big Ben. The Tower of London. The Houses of Parliament. But my favourite exhibition was the Guinness World of Records. I'd been given the *Guinness Book of Records* every Christmas, and always read it with increased vigour, hoping one day to have my own name listed.

The museum had a great range of exhibits, but the one that had the biggest impact on me was the Olympics section. Bob Beamon's eight-metre long jump marked out on the floor amazed me. Impossible. Inhuman. Different class. One-day I hoped I'd make it to the Olympics. I could run; I could run forever. I'd be an elite long-distance runner one day, competing for Ireland in the 10,000 metres and the marathon. Probably on the same day.

SUMMER 1988 – ONE YEAR BEFORE THE INJURY

I was always a bit of an entrepreneur. Not quite Del Boy with a Navan accent, but I started my first business at the age of twelve. It was called Moss Poles International. The idea was simple really. Swiss Cheese Plants were quite popular with members of my family at the time. Some people called them Monsteras, but to me they were always just Cheese Plants.

The thing about these plants though, is that they're easy to grow, but difficult to grow with big leaves unless you can provide them with support. And we all need something or someone to lean against from time to time. Me especially. So I founded Moss Pole International to help people grow bigger leaves on their Cheese Plants. Bill Gates I was not.

But while my head was full of bright ideas, my pockets were sadly empty. Because of this, I had to keep my overheads to a minimum. My Grandfather was able to help as he had plenty of rubber pipe tubing that I could use for free. In fact, the only thing I had to buy was fishing wire from Rod and Gun, a tackle supply shop down the road from my house. After that, it was just a matter of foraging for moss around the back fields where Blackwater Park is now. It was labour intensive, but it was free, and every piece of moss meant profit.

Once I'd managed to amass enough, I used the fishing wire to secure the moss to the pole and sold my creations to the local flower shops for £1, making a fortune in the first few weeks.

However, it soon became apparent that I'd made two big mistakes. Cheese Plants were not as popular outside members of my family as I had assumed and, even when people bought them, they are notoriously slow growers, something I had failed to comprehend in my eureka moment earlier that summer. Shortly after, I liquidated the company and decided that next year would be my year.

However, it would be a couple of years before I started my first paid job. Because Sean Cooney knew me from Navan Shamrocks, and knew my potential not just as a casual runner but as someone who wanted to experience organised races, he asked me to come to his garage every Saturday afternoon. I'd sit there patiently, sometimes reading, sometimes just watching everyone going about their business, until the mechanics had finished up for the day.

Once they were done, I'd get to work throwing wooden shavings over the floor to soak up the oil stains. Then I'd sweep it all up and wipe down the countertops. It didn't take long, and Sean would give me £10 once I was finished. With Jonathan Swift burning a hole in my trousers, I'd race to the shop to buy a packet of McVities HobNobs. When I got home, I'd give the change to Mam for the Credit Union and savage the biscuits.

And while you wouldn't consider HobNobs part of the diet of an elite athlete, I was playing so much sport at that stage, I was able to work off my Saturday treat. In addition to football and running, I'd taken to playing rugby with the school. And I loved it after graduating from playing underage with Navan RFC.

I didn't start every game, but when I got my turn I always tried my best. I certainly wasn't one to sulk about not being picked. One day, St, Pats had to go on the road to play Newbridge College. I was stunned to hear that I'd been picked to play with the juniors. But I was also terrified because I was only 14 and suddenly I'd be going up against these massive 16 and 17 year olds. I don't know how I didn't get sick on the way down. I just kept thinking about something Dad had told me before, 'take them low, Philip. Tap tackle the fuckers.'

Once we arrived, however, I found out I'd been demoted to the second year team. I wasn't sure if I should be angry, happy, disappointed, or all three. But I was still a competitor, I used the chip on my shoulder as motivation and played out of my skin at scrum half that day. I was all over the pitch and I don't think the back line got much of the ball because I wanted to win it myself.

I scored tries, I kicked conversions. I even took a lineout throw myself because I wanted to be Pierre Berbizier in a St Pat's jersey. Thankfully the prop popped it straight back to me and I darted over the line for a classic try.

I was brilliant that day.

I was unstoppable.

CHAPTER 4

FROM THE CONTENDER TO THE BRAWL

26 NOVEMBER 1989 – FIVE HOURS AFTER THE INJURY

I was on the 5 to 10pm shift in Navan Hospital. I'd only walked in the door and was told to report to casualty as there was a transfer to Beaumont Hospital in Dublin. When I went in I could see it was Philip. I knew it was him because I recognised his mother from Chislers, the boutique she worked in.

At first, he was conscious, coherent, and chatting. He knew his name, knew he'd had an accident, and the ambulance was ready to take him to Beaumont.

We left Navan hospital some time between 5:30 and 6pm. Initially, Philip was quite chatty, but as the journey progressed he deteriorated somewhat and eventually slipped into unconsciousness. There was a doctor with me in the ambulance. But he was new. Only an intern. And he was really just travelling with us to tick a box.

But now Philip had stopped responding. He was not just unconscious, but he was having a number of seizure-like episodes in the ambulance. I knew that time was of the essence at that stage and that we needed to get there very fast.

From the moment Philip went unconscious, there was a mad rush to Beaumont. It was like lightning the whole way. The ambulance driver was Pat Brady. Even with his driving, it would have taken at least an hour to get there because there were no motorways back then.

By the time we got to Beaumont, Philip was quite ill. He was immediately rushed into the main resuscitation area and there was a team of doctors there in seconds surrounding him. But we didn't put him on a ventilator.

I don't know why we didn't put him on a ventilator straight away.

Bridie Fitzsimons, nurse who accompanied Phil to Beaumont Hospital

JANUARY 1990 – SIX WEEKS AFTER THE INJURY

I'm like a newborn baby. I can't walk. I can't talk. I can't even eat. I'm being fed through a nasogastric tube shoved up my nose and down my throat. I hate it. I've pulled it out a few times but everyone gets annoyed with me when I do. Still, I can't stand the feeling of it against my throat. They're telling me I can have real food soon. Well, real food so long as it comes in liquid or pureed form. All I want is Corn Flakes, but when I told the nurse she physically recoiled. 'You can't do that Philip, it will be like eating razor blades. You haven't used your throat in months, you have to build up to that sort of food,' she said.

Months. Months of remembering little or nothing, and what I do remember I can't even trust. I have certain memories of being in a coma, but I don't know how much of it is real or how much I dreamed. I can see my Mam and Dad at my bedside showing me pictures of Lucky, my faithful dog. I can feel my sister rubbing my feet, trying to stave off the spasticity the doctors have warned could set in. And that's about it. I don't even really remember one visitor who caused lots of sideways glances and open-mouthed looks when he showed up in ICU with a cowboy hat. It turned out he was a representative of Rutgers American football team, and hand-delivered a signed football ahead of their game in Lansdowne Road. Word had reached the team that I had been due to attend the game, but couldn't because of the incident.

When I did eventually wake up, I believed everything they told me about the previous six weeks. I mean, I had to, I had no other choice.

When my mind drifts off, I have broken fragments of the day of the injury too, but I can no longer tell if they're my memories or those of other people who were there. I can see myself wandering aimlessly around the pitch, the fog in my head compounding the fog in the air. Suddenly I'm sitting in a dugout. My head is sore, but I'm too tired to care. Someone is stabbing the back of my head with something sharp. But I'm so sleepy.

The next thing I know, I'm slowly waking up in a strange room as Sinead O'Connor's 'Nothing Compares to You' is playing in the background. I try to talk, but I can't, with the combination of aphasia and that damned tube down the back of my neck.

I have to use an alphabet board to communicate. It's a great solution, but it's so, so slow. Thankfully, it only took a few hastily spelled 'I ... W ... A ... N ... T ... T ... O ... G ... O ... T ... O ... T ... H ... E ... T ... O ... I ...' before Mam and the nurses realised a bedpan would be needed and quickly,

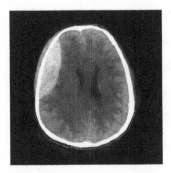

Sketch of CT scan of Phil's brain, by Cintia Roma de Freitas and Dr Jonathan McNulty, from the CT scan report.

after I took too long to spell it the first time. I didn't know it then, but this was probably the first part of my rehabilitation, with the neuropsychologist wanting to see if and how I could communicate.

I wouldn't admit this to anyone, but I've been a terrible patient. I'm fine when Mam or Dad are here, or even my friends and family, but I've reached the point where I want someone with me the whole time. I don't want to be alone. I don't want to have these jigsaw thoughts and nobody there to help me piece them together. It's not so bad now, there's usually somebody around. But I've been isolated in a private room because I've contracted MRSA. Nobody bothered to tell me this was why, but I read it in my file. Mam didn't know either when I said it to her.

When I am on my own, the only thing keeping me going is my Commodore 64. The joystick is a little hard to control because I don't have very much feeling in my right hand at this moment, thanks to the paralysis all the way down that side of my body. The doctors tell me it's called hemiplegia, and they're as uncertain as to whether it will go away as I am of spelling it. To play the Commodore 64, I have to pull myself up from a lying position with my right hand. The physios don't like it when I do this though; they say I'm not ready to put that sort of pressure on that part of my body. But I look at it as rehab. The joystick is a great way of rehabbing my writing hand.

Pac Man, Aztec Challenge, Boulder Dash, Bubble Bobble, Knight Rider, Karate Kid, Paperboy, Question of Sport, Robocop, Winter Games, Wonderboy, Terminator, etc, are also great for testing my brain function. At least that's what I tell Mam the doctors say to when she gives out to me for spending too much time on the computer. But it's true. They're happier now that I'm pressing the button on the joystick rather than constantly pushing my alarm button with some fake request or another designed to ensure someone would be in the room with me.

Even though I can't play sports right now, I'm still finding ways to make it part of my life. Whether it is competing against the guest athletes on 'A Question of Sport', or coaching Ireland during the rugby or football matches that popped up periodically. I've noticed something different though. During live sport in particular, I find it really hard to keep my concentration, drifting off to sleep more often than not. The tiredness in general is overwhelming. Even though I crave company, when visitors make their way to my room I often fall asleep before they leave.

It has mostly been family so far. A few mates have popped in every now and again, but they're studying for the mocks and getting to Beaumont from Navan isn't the easiest thing in the world for a 15 year old. I don't see that though. Instead I tell myself that they don't want to visit me. Why would they want to see me, my body battered and my brain broken?

I won't tell anyone, but it does hurt me that nobody from the football team has come to see me. Mam says that maybe they can't deal with what happened. That there are all sorts of mad stories going around that I'm still in a coma, or that I've been left as a vegetable. They've never had to deal with anybody they knew with such a potentially profound disability. But I can tell from her voice that there was something else too. That maybe they couldn't deal with how they laughed as I stumbled around the pitch and fell asleep in the dugout and felt guilty now for laughing?

But I still wanted to see them. And when I didn't, I got as frustrated as I did when other things didn't go my way. My brain has changed. I've no filter, regularly coming out with inappropriate comments that would disgust or amuse my visitors. Normally they were about Darryl Hannah in *Splash*.

Frustratingly, I can't control my emotions. Simple things, things other people don't even notice are driving me mad. A sneeze in the room next door sent me into a sulk the other day. And I've lost count of the number of times I've cried because somebody opened the door of my room too quickly.

In the odd moments that I am content to be left alone with my thoughts, I use the time to consider just how strange everything is now. Yes, it's weird that I can no longer use my legs after dreaming of racing Kenyans at the Olympics. But I've also lost the ability to cough. I've had two chest infections and a bout of pneumonia and my chest is full of phlegm that I can't clear. They had to suction it out recently and I don't want to repeat that experience again any time soon. The noise of the machine was awful to listen to and Mam had to leave the room as it sucked all the gunk from my lungs. However, the relief I've felt since has made the trauma of the procedure worth it.

Other than Mam, my most regular visitors are the surgeon's team but they rarely speak to me about my condition. Instead, they talk over my bed to Mam as if I don't exist; a ventriloquist's dummy cast aside because the grown ups are talking now. I'll never say it, of course, but it probably does make sense they're talking to Mam. All that medical jargon wouldn't have meant much to me even if my brain was in full working order. What I do hear constantly though is 'two years.' I assume this means I'll be back up and running at full fitness in two years. It seems a long way away but I'll take it right now. And I've always wanted to run a marathon, what better occasion than my 18th birthday?

Two years, I can handle two years. Especially as the doctors mentioned I might be getting home in a few weeks.

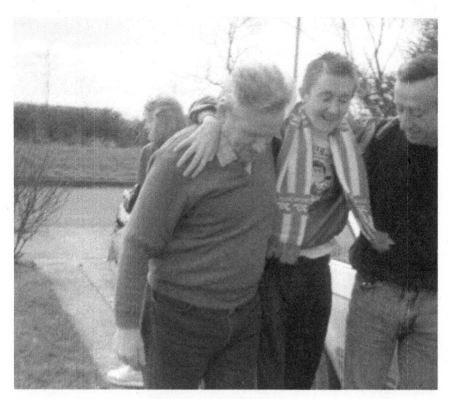

Being carried into our house for the first time, after four months in Beaumont Hospital. My dog, Lucky, didn't forget me and never left my lap when I was placed in the chair.

MARCH 1990 – FOUR MONTHS AFTER THE INJURY

To get home, I had to be carried into 67a, because my legs wouldn't keep me up just yet. Lucky, my faithful terrier, is ecstatic to see me. Four months is about five years in dog years. He won't stop licking the face off me. Even now, as I'm settled into an armchair, he's up on my lap and refusing to move.

There won't be a bed available in Dún Laoghaire for a few weeks yet, so I'm here for a bit. I'm nervous about it though. Days like today are great, when the house is full to the brim with visitors and we can't keep the kitchen stocked with tea and biscuits. These days are fine. It's the physio I'm not looking forward to. Pushing myself when deep down I'm still terrified the next fall is going to be the one that sends me back to Beaumont. Mam and Dad are great, of course, but they've wrapped me so tightly in cotton wool I'm not quite sure how I'm going to escape.

Still, I can tell they're delighted to have me here. Even if they must be absolutely terrified with the hand they'd been dealt. Sure, they have their eldest son home after three months in hospital. And it's great that he's back from the brink after being given a 25% chance to live. But on the other hand, none of us have any idea what the future holds. I thought I'd be walking properly by now, but I'm not. We've no idea if the rehabilitation in Dún Laoghaire is going to work either. They're talking about moving to somewhere more suitable in the centre of town, but I know they can't afford it. We never go without love, food, shelter and everything that a family should have of course, and we always get smashing birthday and Christmas presents, but I hope they don't stretch themselves just for me. Not when we've no idea what the future holds.

It doesn't help that my mood swings are getting worse. I can't help it though. Have you any idea how frustrating it is to have the emotions of a sixteen-year-old trapped in the body of a six-month-old? My siblings have already started to distance themselves as much as they can from me. They have their own friends, their own lives to get on with. They don't need their cripple brother dragging them down. I used to be able to play with them from dusk to dawn. Now I can't even put a spoon to my mouth without getting half of the contents all over my face. I feel like a shadow of myself. A twisted, broken shadow. I thought I'd be happy to be home, but now I just want everyone to go away.

It's time for bed. And even though I know this space so well, I'm still a little uncertain of myself. I know I should be trying to walk. Instead, I crawl around the house on my hands and knees. I've lost all confidence in my ability to stay upright. I just keep thinking about falling.

In my dreams that night, I'm still able-bodied. I'm running the length of Kalungwishi Street, chasing down John Ngugi, Dieter Baumann and Hansjörg Kunze for an Olympic medal.

But when I wake I'm disabled again.

CHAPTER 5

I'M STILL STANDING

26 NOVEMBER 1989 – TWO HOURS AFTER THE INJURY

Medical notes of Philip Quinlan

MAY 1990 – SEVEN MONTHS AFTER THE INJURY

I feel like I'm stumbling around in a fog, waiting to be swallowed whole by the shadows. The only thing I feel is fear. Fear of the pain getting worse. Fear of the pain never going away. Fear of never playing football again. Never running again. Never being me again.

And nobody understands. Nobody gets it. I didn't ask for this. I didn't choose this. I'm sitting outside the principal's office now because I've stood up to the bullies. The teacher just doesn't understand that I can only talk in a whisper they can't hear. Or doesn't care.

They look at me with sympathy because they know I've been through something, but they talk to me as if I'm stupid sometimes. Who knows, maybe I'd have ended up sitting here a few more times if I was fully functional? Imagine me, in trouble for running too fast in the hallways. But now they've realised it takes me so long to get my bag and walk out the door that it's not worth the effort of sending me to sit outside Mr Kennedy's office.

A couple of my classmates walk by. Eyes down. They don't understand either. What's their problem? Are they embarrassed to know me? Are they worried they're going to catch the disability off me if I stand too close to them? I'm not cool anymore; I can't join in when they're talking about the match at the weekend or their new personal best for the 1500 metres. Maybe they're just jealous that I can wear runners because of my rough, plastic splint, while they're stuck in their poxy shoes all day.

The truth, of course, is not something I can know just yet, not something that my brain will process until I'm much older. They're probably just as confused as me by the suddenness of it all, and they feel awkward and nervous of saying the wrong thing. But I can't know these things. I'm too young.

What I do know is pain. My ingrown toenails are a constant source. I've bandaged the big toe on my right foot to help keep some of the agony at bay, but it only works for a short while. I can't even change my gait to take the pressure off. So I'm stuck with the pain, just like I'm stuck here, waiting to hear the principal tell me he's not angry at me for standing up to my bullies, just disappointed. Expecting that same look of pity on his face again.

Don't get me wrong, it is great to get back to the structure of school and to see my friends. I was especially excited the first morning, when my best friend Ken and his Dad, Patsy, collected me to go to school. Patsy, a science teacher in St Pat's and ever the joker, looked back in the car and said with a smile, 'I hope you have your homework done!' Ken was always watching out for me in school. He always stopped in the corridors to ask me if I was ok. He'd tell all the other popular guys that I was alright. At home, he'd invite me into his house regularly so we could just hang out. Ken always had patience for me.

But the endless walking of corridors is exhausting – every forty minutes, going from class to class, while trying to dodge the lads who would try to push me over or, worse still, mimic my limp for their own entertainment. And while I know all this walking is a form of physio that will be very beneficial, I know deep down that it's not going to get me back to full health. Maybe that's why I take the slings and arrows so personally.

But, God, I've grown to fucking despise asking for help. I don't want anyone to see me as a burden. I'm too proud. And yet I know I'm a massive hypocrite too. I've learned to love nothing more than when people do something spontaneous for me. But I've become so quick to say no that people have just stopped asking.

This isn't how it's supposed to be. This isn't how it's supposed to be at all. This wasn't how rehabilitation was. In fact, the only reason I'm back in school at all is because Dún Laoghaire was so good for me. If people ask about my rehab there, I tell them how much I loved it. Because I really did. So much of my rehabilitation was based around sport that I took to it like a Phil to water.

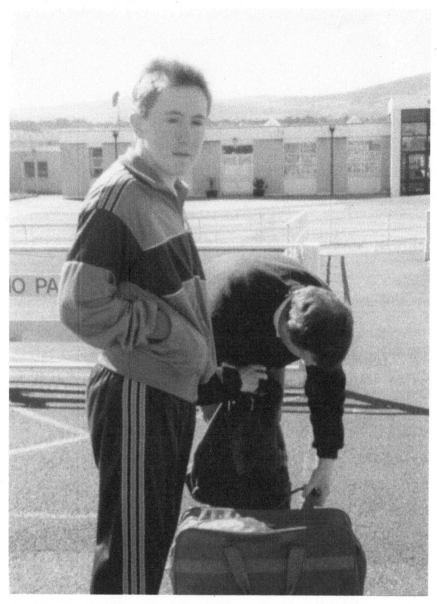

Going back to the Rehabilitation Centre in Dún Laoghaire for more intense physio, which would allow me go back to school in September.

I wasn't so sure on the first day we arrived, as we struggled to find the building. But as Mam and Dad waited in the lobby area, I wobbled off down the corridor, finding the sports hall after thirty minutes of painfully slow shuffling. The pool table was the first thing I spotted, not knowing how much time I was going to spend hanging around that particular spot over the next few months.

Mam found me and helped me to my bed and, after making sure I was settled, they both said their goodbyes. They seemed upset. But I was well used to wards and being prodded and poked at this stage, so I didn't feel nervous at all.

The first thing I noticed was how well everyone got on. How easy it was just to chat to people. Much more so than with my school friends. I suppose it's because we were all in the same boat, even if the oceans we were trying to cross were worlds apart.

There was the fellah who'd been in a car crash in Limerick and who hadn't left the bed in thirteen years. 'He's probably still there now,' I think to myself, looking up at the clock and wondering how long it'll be before I'm called into Mr Kennedy.

I laugh when I think of Paddy Carroll, who was in the bed next to mine and whose pitch got higher and higher the more excited or angry he got. We hit it off straight away. Paddy was a lot older than me. But he'd had a stroke, which meant he was enduring intense rehab too. He understood what I was going through, and was like a surrogate big brother to me.

'He still owes me that £20,' I suddenly remember. He bet me that I couldn't get Una, the impossibly pretty student nurse from Dublin, to kiss me. There aren't many girls like Una in school. There aren't many girls like Una anywhere.

Because he got to go home at weekends, Paddy didn't make the trip to see *Cats* in Dublin, but a lot of us did. As much as I loved Dún Laoghaire, it was great to get out for a bit. Those of us who could loaded up, slowly, onto the bus that would bring us to The Point.

We were paired up to make sure nobody wandered off, and my partner was a blind guy who was, again, slightly older than me. But he was funny, and we chatted the whole way into town. I loved every minute of the show and at the end, he turned to me and said, 'That was the best thing I've ever seen.'

And I saw the look on his face. The projection of bravado. The look of someone who didn't take himself or his condition too seriously. I swore at that moment that I wouldn't take myself too seriously either, but the looks and words of other people constantly put me on the defensive. I could joke about my condition, but nobody else could.

Maybe that's why I'm struggling to settle back into school. All the men I made friends with in Dún Laoghaire were just that: men. They had so much life experience that I'd often just sit in silence, listening as they spoke. While my friends back in Navan were worried about whether they'd get the shift at the next school disco, these men had lived. They'd seen the world. They'd got their shift. They made me realise that there was so much I didn't know, and so much I wanted to see and do. That made the actual rehabilitation so much easier to endure.

It's a good thing too, because physio was on my schedule every day. Sometimes twice or three times a day. It was exhausting. But, because I was so competitive, I revelled in trying to beat my own personal bests in the various tasks set by Ann O'Brien, one of the senior therapists. She was trying to give me back control of my body. I was trying to walk fifty metres, unaided, in ten minutes or less.

Even though my right leg was the most obvious sign of the injury, a huge part of Ann's recovery plan focused on my right arm. As an orthodox puncher, there was a lot of work needed to get some semblance of normality back into the arm. It was never going to get back to what it was – that ship had sailed – but I needed to be able to hold a pen and write if I wanted to get back to school.

Sitting here, I'm almost sorry I did so well.

The evenings in Dún Laoghaire were the best part. We got to spend all our time in the sports hall, at various events and competitions. Basketball games were the most competitive, and the families even got involved. I remember my brother James having to jump into a wheelchair to make up the numbers and compete against those who actually needed wheelchairs.

It was a brilliant laugh, but ultra-competitive. The atmosphere around the place was uplifting, so inspiring compared to the shite I'm having to put up with in school.

But I know now that the relief it brought was an imposter. A tease. I know all too clearly that it only visits for a short while. It's a trespasser. I'm far more comfortable dealing with chronic pain. It's more reliable. It doesn't pretend to be anything it's not.

Not like me.

Sitting here pretending I'm okay, when all I can think is, 'What doesn't kill you sometimes makes you wish it had.'

CHAPTER 6

AND A BANG ON THE EAR

26 NOVEMBER 1989 – FIVE HOURS AFTER THE INJURY

I remember getting ready for the cycle to the game, but my Dad said he'd drive me up instead. The fog was too bad to cycle in, he reckoned. So bad the game would probably be called off anyway. In fact, he was certain it would be when we arrived and the fog was much thicker in Kilberry than it had been in Navan.

The referee arrived and we lost our minds laughing at him. He pulled up on this old red-and-white Honda 50, wearing these big thick black wellies. Dad grabbed him and asked him if he was going to let us get home before the fog got even worse, but he shrugged him off and never bothered to answer him.

At points during the game, you couldn't see more than fifteen metres or so ahead of you. You'd send a pass across the field and have no idea whether it got to one of our lads or one of theirs. Two minutes into the game, the Parkvilla keeper kicked the ball out and it just appeared out of the mist and landed between me and Gordon Mitchell. We looked at other with an expression that said, 'What the fuck?' I passed the ball on, but to who, I've no clue.

The next thing I remember is both Philip and Ray jumping for a ball about ten metres in front of me at the Torro end of the field, almost in line with their dugout. Initially it looked as if Ray had come off a little worse. I'd played football and rugby with Philip for years and knew he was a hardy little lad, so I wasn't at all surprised to see him run it off.

It wasn't really until half-time and Philip was sitting in the dugout that it all went downhill fast. But even then, as we played the second half in almost total darkness, I don't think anyone thought it was going to be any worse than a headache and a bandage.

That said, as we drove home, I could tell Dad was worried. He'd worked in the mines, and he'd seen some of the effects of head injuries before. The drive home was horrendous because of the fog, it was almost impossible to see. When we got back, he told me to run around to Philip's house straight away and see if there was any update.

As I went to leave, Philip's sister was at the door, asking what happened. It wasn't until later that evening she was able to tell us just how bad it was, and that Philip was fighting for his life.

That evening, as I sat in my room, I fell out of love with football. And I never played another game, not for Torro or any other team.

Donal Greene, ex-Torro United player

26 NOVEMBER – THE MOMENT OF THE INJURY

Dad drops me to the Round O carpark at 1.15pm. I'd normally cycle, but he insists today that he'll bring me. The drive is quiet, even for Dad. I'm not sure if he's volunteered to be a taxi because of the fog or because he's worried I wouldn't go otherwise. To be honest, I'm not feeling great. It's probably just a head cold, not the sort of thing that would normally stop me playing. But combined with the weather, I've little interest in togging out.

We get to the car park, and Kerr Reilly's bus is waiting to take us to the gate beside the haystack shed. That's as far as it can go, but we're all well used to walking across the two fields from there to to the pitch. As we get ready on the side of the pitch, the lads are still laughing at the referee turning up in his wellies on a Honda 50.

I can just about make out some of the Torro lads warming up on the other sideline. Donal Greene is there; so's Ray Kealy. I'm surprised at that. Liverpool are playing Arsenal this afternoon, surely Ray wouldn't want to miss that. Mind you, if you were to listen to the Torro players in school this week, you'd swear this was their FA Cup final. Maybe that's why he didn't want to miss it: bragging rights.

'Brazil,' I think to myself, making a note to remind Ray after the game that I want my Subbuteo team back. For ages he only had Shamrock Rovers, and there's only so often you can play five on five Rovers versus Celtic on a full-size Subbuteo pitch. Still, it's not as bad as Trev and his blue tablecloth for a pitch. Sometimes I wonder if the lads take Subbuteo seriously enough at all.

We start the game slowly enough. We're used to beating teams by eight or nine goals. But the fog is getting worse. It's impossible to see the far side of the pitch if you're hugging the touchline. We score; Liam Carey got it. As we're celebrating, he tells us he beat five players, rounded the keeper twice and then scored. But it could just as easily have been a one-yard tap-in for all I can tell.

The fog is getting worse now, and it's cold. I knew I should have stayed in bed. Mind you, at least I'm pretending to give a shite. Neville Dunne over there might as well have left his jeans and farmer's hat on for all the running he's doing.

I get possession a couple of times and try to find a team-mate, but it's a lottery where the ball might end up. The worst are the kick-outs though. One might hit you a bang on the ear before you even realised the ball was coming your direction.

The ball goes out of play, and the ref says there are fifteen minutes to go to half-time. I think to myself that maybe, if we grab another couple, he might just tell us all to go home then. We're clearly the better team, and he gets paid that way regardless.

'Quinno, to you!' a shout rings out from the fog. And sure enough, the ball is bouncing head-height between myself and Ray. I get my head in first and flick the ball on, just in time for Ray's head to collide with the back of mine. Crack.

26 NOVEMBER 26 – ONE MINUTE AFTER THE INJURY

'Are you alright, son?' asks the referee after I've had the magic sponge applied by the manager.

'Yeah, it wasn't that bad,' I say, rubbing the back of my ear.

'Do you know where you are?'

'I do, of course. I'm in Kilberry.'

'What day is it?'

'Sunday.'

'How many fingers am I holding up?'

'Three.'

'Okay. You're grand.'

26 NOVEMBER – FIVE MINUTES AFTER THE INJURY

The fog is getting much worse.

It's a lot harder to see now.

Jesus, he's going to have to call this game off. I can't see a ...

'Quinno, would you pay attention? That ball was there to be won,' comes a roar from the dugout.

I spin round, I don't see the ball, but the world keeps spinning after I stop.

I think I'm going to be sick.

26 NOVEMBER – TEN MINUTES AFTER THE INJURY

Half-time at last. I'm so tired.

'Quinno, you're coming off,' says Gerry Browne, the manager.

Normally I'd complain. But I'm exhausted.

'Ha ha, Philip's fallen asleep,' I hear one of the lads say as he shakes my shoulder. There's lots of laughter.

'Oh fuck, there's blood coming from his ear.'

26 NOVEMBER – TWENTY MINUTES AFTER THE INJURY

'Kerr, get the bus ready!' I hear Gerry scream. But he sounds like he's down a tunnel.

I'm so sore now. It feels like someone was beating me black and blue in the dugout.

Was today a rugby game?

No, it couldn't be. It was football. We were playing ... who were we playing again?

26 NOVEMBER – THIRTY MINUTES AFTER THE INJURY

I'm being carried shoulder-height by the lads. We must have won the World Cup. Did I score?

There's Kerr Reilly's minibus. How did he get that to Stadio Olimpico? He complains about having to drive to Slane.

He's screaming at me not to go to sleep. It's the last thing I hear before I doze off again.

26 NOVEMBER – NINETY MINUTES AFTER THE INJURY

I'm climbing trees at 151 Kalungwishi Street. I'm not sure how I got back here, but the weather has taken a nice turn.

I fall.

There are nurses everywhere now. Kerr is shouting at someone to take a look at me.

I look at the floor. Is that blood? Black blood?

Is that my black blood?

My grandad arrives from his house close by.

I ask him, 'Am I going to die?'

26 NOVEMBER – THREE HOURS AFTER THE INJURY

'You're in an ambulance, Philip, it's okay.'

I haven't even asked. But I must look confused.

I've no idea who is talking to me.

I'm tired. My head hurts.

26 NOVEMBER – FIVE HOURS AFTER THE INJURY

I can hear my uncle Dave talking to Liz, my aunt. He's a heart surgeon. Maybe he's here to help me?

'The CT scan shows a large bleed on the right side, pushing the brain over to the left-hand side.

'But the worst thing is that the upper part of the brain is being shoved down through a narrow part inside of the skull, which is extraordinarily dangerous.

'It looks like it may be fatal.'

27 NOVEMBER – ONE DAY AFTER THE INJURY

It's uncle Dave again. He must have helped them fix me.

'Things look a little better, but still serious.

'I would be worried about the outlook.'

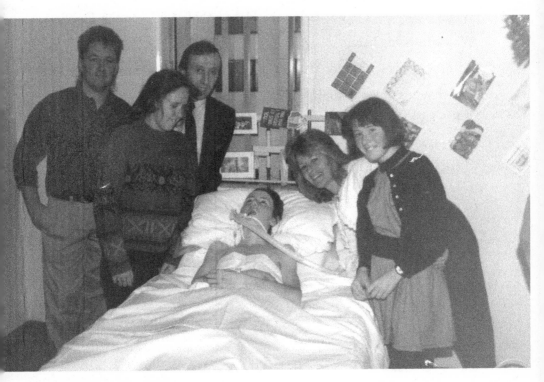

Christmas Day 1989.

3 DECEMBER 1989 – ONE WEEK AFTER THE INJURY

I can't believe I'm getting to run alongside Eamonn Coghlan. And at the Olympics.

When was the last time Ireland had two men in the final of the 5000 metres? Probably never.

He's older now. I can definitely take him. But if we want to get near the Kenyans, we're going to have to work together.

We nod at the start line. The plan is clear. We need to slow the whole thing right down. If the pace is too fast, they'll beat us easily. Hold them up. Kick for the line with 600 metres to go and we'll have a chance.

I wave to Colm O'Rourke in the crowd. Jack Charlton's there too. There's Willie Anderson. He was facing the Haka only last weekend in Dublin. What's he doing here?

The race has started and Sean Cooney from Navan Shamrocks is track-side, shouting at me to run.

But I can't move.

My legs won't work.

Why won't my legs work?

CHAPTER 7

BABY WE WERE BORN TO RUN

30 APRIL 1990 – FIVE MONTHS AFTER THE INJURY

I have reviewed Philip in the neurological clinic today and I must say I am very impressed by the great progress he has been making. Considering the very severe nature of his head injury he has done exceptionally well. He has good motivation, seems to be in very good spirits and there are no obvious problems with concentration, memory, abstract thought etc. Physically of course he does have right sided dyspraxia and weakness but he is working extremely hard at this and he is young enough to improve much more.

I note that they are contemplating a return to school in September and I would have thought that it is very important before this to get a formal psychological assessment. This would pinpoint any particular problems, say with language or numeracy, which could perhaps be worked on before he returns. I have written to Martina O'Connor our Clinical Psychologist asking her if she would arrange this.

I'll see him again myself in about four months.

Steven Young, Consultant Neurosurgeon

SUMMER 1992 – THREE YEARS AFTER THE INJURY

My grandfather was a bus conductor on the Dublin–Edenderry route, so it was always destined that I'd travel. It was in the genes. The summer of 1992 saw my first big trip away after the injury. I had decided to volunteer with l'Arche, a French community for people with intellectual disabilities. It was, of course, just a happy coincidence that three months in France would help with my French oral for the Leaving the following year.

Mam was a bit worried about the whole thing, but herself and my godfather Robby dropped me to the Gare de Nord in Paris for my onward journey to Compiègne, north of Paris. A bus then brought me to Trosly Breuil, where l'Arche is located. I was wandering around, quite lost, when a young lady spotted me and asked if I needed a lift anywhere. She was either very brave or very stupid to be picking up a stranger – or maybe I was for getting into a stranger's car – but she told me she knew where l'Arche was located and offered to bring me. Maybe she thought I was part of the special needs community she lived close to!

We did our best to communicate during the short trip in her fire-engine-red Citroën Dyane, me in broken Navan French and her in scattered Oise English. She gave me her number and made me promise to phone her when I got settled. She kissed me as we said goodbye, and I really didn't want to leave the car.

After a couple of days at l'Arche, I was sorry I did. The French I'd learned in school and the language spoken in the real world were oceans apart. But it didn't take long for my confidence to grow. By day three, I was enjoying speaking and hearing the language as much as I was the work of engaging with the intellectually disabled people in the centre.

On that third night, I made a life-changing decision. I binned my entire prescription of Epanutin. It had been part of my life for over two years, prescribed to halt the seizures I'd taken while unconscious at Beaumont Hospital. I had hundreds of seizures in the early days, most of which, thankfully, I can't remember. I was either in the coma or unconscious. Mam was terrified every time I took a seizure, and had escalated the matter with the medical team in Beaumont to review my meds.

Although this was the first time I'd been away by myself, I knew my own body and head better than the surgeons, and surely the drugs were only a precaution? I'd been on them for over two years now and the only incident I'd had was when I went to the Beechmount Hotel nightclub for the first time. I saw stars, and my eyes took about half an hour to readjust. Thankfully I had lots of friends there. The strobe lights weren't very kind to my eyes, and by extension, my brain. John Travolta and the Bee Gees were safe from another contender.

But away from the bright lights, in my tiny room in l'Arche, I made the very conscious decision to dump the drugs. In my heart, I knew weaning myself off the Epanutin was probably better, but I wanted to go cold turkey. These drugs had been a cumbersome routine ever since returning home to Navan. Most mornings, over breakfast, I'd remember to take them before heading off to school. Some mornings I'd forget, but Mam and Dad would always ask if I'd 'taken my pill'. I didn't like this line of questioning at all. I knew they were only asking out of concern, but I didn't want them to have this responsibility too. They'd done enough.

But what really made my mind up was that this felt like a new beginning. I wanted the previous chapter of my life finished, and fuck the consequences. So I dumped them, *dans la poubelle*.

That night, I dreamed about running again.

Over the next couple of days, everything was going well in l'Arche until more volunteers arrived to work alongside us. I was told I was no longer going to work directly with people with intellectual disabilities. For the next four weeks, or maybe more, I'd be based in a workshop, folding leaflets for a summer promotion. But I hadn't come to France to fold leaflets in a damp outhouse, so I hijacked my way out of the place.

I phoned Amelie, who kindly came to collect me. After spending the night at her place, she dropped me to the train station in Compiegne and, a little over a week after departing from there, I returned to Gare de Nord. There was no Mam or Robby there to collect me though. I was young, single and relatively free, and determined to make the most of my time in Paris.

Amelie had helped me to find accommodation, but instead of taking the Métro to my accommodation, I decided to prove myself by walking. I dragged my suitcase *sur les routes et boulevards*, sweat pouring from me from the effort. My French was good enough that I was comfortable stopping strangers to ask: *Où est Rue de Mouffetard?* Three hours, two buckets of sweat and one scabby old *Rough Guide to Paris* later, I found my hostel.

After resting up for a few hours, I decided to take in some of the Parisian nightlife. I wobbled to the nearest Métro station and made my way to the Franklin D Roosevelt stop. It was some challenge to negotiate the Métro at first, but I soon became quite adept and learned to enjoy the experience. I walked the length of the Avenue des Champs-Élysées and onwards to Place de la Concorde, savouring all of the sights and sounds. Making my way along the Rue de Rivoli, I remembered watching Tour de France finishes down through the years.

The LeMond/Fignon time trial was racing through my mind as I wobbled over to the Louvre. I was let in without a *billet*, maybe because I was Irish. Or maybe it was because I was disabled. I took my time visiting all the rooms, and finally got to see the Mona Lisa. In the presence of her greatness, I decided I could live in Paris. I'd only been here a day, but I'd fallen in love with the city.

The real highlight was Montmartre. Climbing to the top of Sacre Coeur was like a finishing line of sorts for me.

During the early days of beginning to wake up, I knew from listening to my parents and the doctors that they all thought there was no chance of my ever doing this sort of travel on my own. Maybe, if I was well enough, they could take me to Euro Disney in a wheelchair and push me around for a few days. 'Ahh, bless him.' They'd have to take me everywhere for the rest of their lives.

Now, standing at the top of Sacre Coeur, all I could think was, 'Fuck me, I'm actually here.' Sure, I'd never climb Machu Picchu or compete in the Hawaii Ironman like I'd promised myself a few years ago. But the fact that I now knew I was mentally and physically capable of doing this by myself was hugely invigorating. Not even my fully able-bodied peers had travelled abroad solo. It felt, for the first time in a couple of years, that I was actually living. And now, across a Parisian canvas, endless travel possibilities spread out in front of me, each painted with as much flourish and care as Leonardo da Vinci used when capturing Lisa Gherardini all those years ago. Given a twenty-five percent chance of living just a few years ago and now here I was with the world at my feet. On my own. Solo.

'You've done it, Quinlan,' I said to myself. 'You've done it.'

NOVEMBER 1995 – SIX YEARS AFTER THE INJURY

My working life began in the local library in Navan in 1995. I've always been a devourer of books, so I adored this work, even if it came with a temporary contract that could be rescinded at any time. I loved the customers – all the elderly ladies used to come in to show off their blue rinse. The ephemeral nature of the job didn't bother me too much, but Dad wasn't sure. Of course, like any father, he was happy to see me working and held out hope that it would turn into something permanent and pensionable. It's what was important back in his day. It has become even more important nowadays. That's all a Dad wants for his disabled son. So it was difficult for me to tell him less than a year later that I'd be leaving. Leaving to work in a special needs summer camp in New Jersey.

My first real job wouldn't come until two years later. Philip 'I work in Banking don't you know' Quinlan. A proper job. A grown up.

Getting off the bus at Busáras, I made it outside to the taxi rank and knew I wasn't a million miles from where I needed to be. But I didn't want to arrive on the first day all sweaty. Once comfortably inside the first car in the rank, I asked the driver to take me to Ulster Bank HQ, just across the Liffey.

He was disgusted.

'Sure you can fucking walk there!'

'I'm disabled!'

He reluctantly pulled off, giving out shite under his breath all the way.

'Fucking waiting on the rank ages and I have to fucking drive this spastic cunt three minutes away. I'll have to go back to join the end of the fucking rank now. Waste of fucking time …'

I got out and he nearly bloody hit me with the £1 tip I gave him.

I was little more than a porter with Ulster Bank, but I enjoyed the work. If I didn't have the injury, postman is a job I definitely could have seen myself doing. Early mornings are when I'm best. But you can't live your life in the *modh coinníollach*, and so I took what I was given.

It seemed that I was determined to work only for high-profile brands, and Aer Lingus came calling after I'd flown through an aptitude test. They offered me a job working in their accounts payable department. But from day one, I felt like an imposter. Everybody looked at me differently. Everyone treated me differently. You could see it in their faces, they were all disgusted by my limp. I was bullied, no two ways about it.

A couple of months in, I came up with what I thought was a better process of doing some accounting. 'We've done it this way for years,' was the comeback. Before I started, I told my parents this was my dream company to work for. I just saw the free travel associated with it. But I was devastated each morning having to get up and go to work. Physically sick. Anxiety central. Any stars in my eyes soon crashed head-first into the sea.

The night I decided I had had enough I was living in a squalid bedsit in Drumcondra, with a dodgy landlord. Everything was so depressing. The job sucked, my home life sucked, so I broke into the bottle of white wine and tried to drown my sorrows. The bottle had been a bedsit-warming present months previously. The next morning, I found out the hard way that sorrows quickly learned to swim and, with the worst hangover of my life, I took the day off to apply for other jobs. Proactive. A month or so later, I was working across the road from Aer Lingus at the Airways Industrial Estate, with Lotus 123.

Lotus was all open-plan, and everybody had access to a desktop computer. I was initially placed in the Nordic Sales team, but sometimes struggled to understand the boss. It was probably her accent. She was, after all, from Dublin. However, my pedantic eye for detail and data-entry skills were much in demand and soon I was asked to lead a new SAP order entry team.

I revelled in dealing with the different characters on the team. Any problem they might have, I'd fix. This working environment was in stark contrast to the outdatedness of Aer Lingus. The vibe was totally different. The Americans did things much better. And they always discussed my ideas and even implemented some of them.

It was a bittersweet time, as I left after a year to travel Down Under. I'd made a lot of friends and the bosses were all very easy to get on with.

After my sojourn to Australia for the Olympics, Lotus were happy to have me back. But despite how much I loved it, it was tough going to get up at 5am for Dad to drop me to the bus to Dublin. When I arrived in town, I'd have to walk from O'Connell Street around to Amiens Street, to another bus that would take me back to the Airways Industrial Estate in Santry. And doing the reverse journey every evening only added to the feeling that this couldn't be a permanent solution.

An apartment was sourced in Phibsboro. Myself and Shane, my Cork compatriot, moved in. I could lie on until 6:30!

However, it was on one of the bus rides back to Navan one Friday evening, that I met a recruitment consultant, who told me they could boost my salary by forty-three percent, from £14,000 to a whopping £20,000 a year, a large sum in those days. After a couple of interviews with Modus Media in Kildare Town, it became clear that they needed me more than I needed them. I told them I was probably going to stick with Lotus 123 until my contract had finished. A month later, I started work with Modus, because they offered me £21,000 a year.

Modus, in turn, sub-contracted me out to Autodesk, where I began my placement as an SAP New Product Introduction Coordinator. A very professional outfit, I learned a lot about the high-paced stresses of this company. I was still sharing an apartment with Shane in Phibsboro and attending a lot of the Bohemians home games in Dalymount Park, just a few hundred metres walk away. It wasn't until a year later that I relocated to Modus headquarters in Kildare Town, while Autodesk migrated to Switzerland.

My pedantic eye for detail made me thrive in this role for five years. The job involved sourcing all the components for Autodesk, abiding by their very strict guidelines. There was little margin for error in producing their design software packages.

We had a fantastic boss, Lillian, who always did more than her fair share. This taught the rest of us to go above and beyond for her. Our small team consisted of Orla and Louise, and worked very well with the very high-maintenance Autodesk customer. It meant a lot of driving to Dublin to pay visits to our vendors and entertain the Autodesk crew whenever they came in from Switzerland.

The last two years with Modus were very disappointing. In my opinion, our team leader had been given a raw deal by the company. She left, to be replaced by someone who, I felt, hadn't the knowledge nor personality to lead a team. I had been offered the job when she was leaving, but turned it down because I'd seen just how much Lillian had given to the role. I wasn't sure I could match her dedication.

LONDON, 1996 – SEVEN YEARS AFTER THE INJURY

I was a very different person to who I was on my previous trip to London a decade earlier, and it was a very different trip. Instead of an organised bus,

I'd hitched a lift in the cab of an articulated lorry bound for Germany, driven by my mate's older brother.

I took the long way to London too, via Bremen and Hamburg to visit a pen pal, so I had to get the bus back to London. This was the first bus I'd ever been on with beds. I was my usual self, talking to whoever had ears. I found myself chatting to another Irishman, Frank from Belfast. He had just arrived in Hamburg after watching his son boxing in the European Championships in Copenhagen.

We struck up a good friendship and I listened to his own stories of boxing years ago. It was good to have this confidant to chat with all along the way. He'd lived through the harshest of the Troubles.

That said, the ferry trip across to Dover wasn't the best, because Frank and I had both only reserved seats. He had a few drinks while I tried my best to sleep. I purposely woke early the following morning, hours before we docked, to spy the famous White Cliffs of Dover. The Cliffs of Moher are far more impressive.

When we arrived in London's Victoria Cross Station, Frank told me he'd leave me in a pub while he went into the bookie's just across the road. Once on a high stool, Frank told the barman to put whatever I had on his tab. I'm not sure anyone knew where to look when I asked for a rock shandy.

Frank went off about his business and I was left talking to the other punters at the bar. One, with a northern Irish accent, told me he'd never been home since he arrived as a teenager. He was too ashamed to set foot back in Ireland after spending his life drinking and working on the buildings. He'd started sending money home years ago, but now everyone was dead. He was almost married, but was left at the altar, never had kids, but was happy alone, with nobody to be accountable to.

He was describing it as a tragedy, but all I could think of was how romantic this sounded. The idea of being the old single uncle, slipping a fiver to his nieces and nephews when he went to visit. Holding court at family funerals and weddings. The mysterious black sheep of the family who wasn't just known for his limp.

A while later, the chap asked me could I help him to the door. Of course I could. He linked my arm and I shuffled with him to the door, opening it and leaving him on the path. It was so unusual to be the support and not the supported for once that it felt a bit like a dream.

But things turned sour very quickly. As he stumbled out the door, my mysterious friend insisted I take five pounds for keeping him company. I refused politely, but suddenly he got very angry and started shouting at me.

'What the fuck is wrong with my money?' he snarled in his Northern Irish accent. 'Not good enough for you, is it?'

He wound up to punch me, but like me, he operated in slow motion. As I stumbled backwards, his fist missed me by a few kilometres.

Frank had spotted my trouble from inside the betting shop window and rushed out to intervene. But it was all over before it really started and, with a couple of words, he ushered my former friend away.

Once we were alone, he produced two fistfuls of fifties. His bet had come up. His payday. We entered the pub again and Frank shadowed me back to the bar, ready to pay for what I had drank. The barman's big pay day hadn't arrived, but I think Frank left a hefty tip in lieu of my extravagant bill.

As we said goodbye, he told me to look out for his son, Damaen, in future bouts. Little did I know he'd be fighting for Ireland in Atlanta that summer. Another Olympian. Always the Olympics.

CHAPTER 8

I WAS UNRECOGNISABLE TO MYSELF

1 DECEMBER 2022 – THIRTY-THREE YEARS AFTER THE INJURY

Specific memories are hazy, but one that stands out – I think it may have been the first day the campers arrived – and we were using the golf buggy to transport luggage around. Phil was enjoying driving the thing and seeing how fast it could go.

We swung around the corner by the main building and there was another vehicle right in front of us, maybe the handyman's pick-up truck. He had to turn sharply to avoid a crash and we went up onto the grass. Our hearts were in our mouths for a second!

But Phil was everyone's best friend at camp. He had a smile or a wink or a story for everyone. If you ever needed to talk about something, Phil was your man. In no time at all his disability became invisible to us. He didn't let it stop him from doing anything.

And that can't have been easy for him chasing all those kids around camp. Phil was just one of the guys with a big personality and an even bigger heart. He left an impression on everyone he met that summer.

Shane O'Driscoll, Camp Merry Heart volunteer

AND A BANG ON THE EAR

JULY 1996 – SEVEN YEARS AFTER THE INJURY

Hackettstown, New Jersey, is the kind of place Bruce Springsteen sings about. Three square miles of battered dreams and broken-down cars. But on 21 O'Brien Road, sepia-tinted images of Americana were left behind as you walked through the gates of Camp Merry Heart. A special needs summer camp, this place was a microcosm of the world. But because we only got to spend three months working there, we had to live our lives in fast-forward.

The process of getting to Merry Heart started in Dublin, on my twenty-second birthday. It had to be an omen. The camp director, Mary Ellen Ross, was intrigued at the idea that I was the eldest of four. I tried flirting with her, and it worked. Or at least I was the last interviewee of the day and she still had one position to fill.

The training also took place in Dublin, fairly basic health-and-safety stuff, in a building on Mountjoy Street. Only two of the three of us who were selected turned up; the third, Nigel, opted instead to escape for a day, on the piss around town.

My sister and her boyfriend dropped us to the airport. Dad wasn't overly impressed that I'd left a good, albeit temporary, job with Meath County Council. Shane, the other volunteer, had travelled from Cork for the experience. There was a little bit of a kerfuffle when my leg splint set off the X-ray machine going through security, but once I pulled up my trousers to show the security guard that it was supporting my leg, I was waved through.

When we got to the other side, there was some class of fancy reception going on. Hostesses were handing out Bucks Fizz. I was feeling particularly wobbly that day, after walking the length of the airport, so I hid my drink beneath my seat in case a sip or two led to a slip or two.

'Excuse me, sir, can you come with me?' a man in uniform said to me. He escorted me to a room off to one side, with a single chair and a TV in the corner. I sat there for ten minutes, wondering what was going on. After ten minutes of sitting on my own, I was invited to board the flight. Shane asked what had happened, but I couldn't answer him. I was just as much in the dark. Did they want to make sure I was able to board the flight safely because of my disability, or were they worried about a drunk Paddy because of the way I walked?

Landing in JFK was awe-inspiring. Overwhelming. A pure adrenaline rush. As we walked through the terminal, Shane and I met Nigel. Little did I know then the huge impact he would have on my life. Orientation would take place in Columbia University, but upon arrival, we just threw our luggage in the bedroom and followed Nigel, disciple-like, to the nearest pizza restaurant. It was my first taste of real pizza, and it was incredible. Nigel and his mates ordered pitchers of beer with straws. I opted against alcohol.

We eventually made our way to Camp Merry Heart, and spent the first week training. We learned what the campers would be like and what disabilities we would encounter, and we learned about the personalities of our fellow counsellors. They had travelled from all over the world to assist the disabled campers, but it was Hana, from the Czech Republic, who caught my eye more than any other. Beautiful. Her English wasn't great, but she was keen to improve and, I soon learned, even keener for me to teach her.

I would be looking after two campers for the first session: Jack, a chronic non-wiper who drove an electric mower (wheelchair), and Norman, who could walk but was severely 'mentally retarded' according to his application form. It turned out that I'd have three campers though, with David joining our trio.

Jack rarely spoke, and when he did it was more whisper than hurricane. What he lacked in vocalisation, however, he made up for in speed in his wheelchair. When Norman arrived, what really struck me was the emptiness in his eyes when we were introduced. I carefully took his hand and led him up towards our cabin.

David was a fantastic bloke, with massive, thick glasses. He had Down Syndrome and, from the moment we met, he really brightened up my day with his infectious humour. The first morning was hectic, but David had to preen himself perfectly. The pride he took in shaving was an eye opener. He folded his pyjamas absolutely seam-perfect, straightened his tie, fixed his glasses, combed his hair and settled his feet into his runners. Ready to go.

As we looked after the campers, so too did we look after ourselves and our burgeoning adulthood. Camp Merry Heart was based around a lake that was abundant with fish. I had my first 'date' with Hana down here with a fishing rod. I caught her a fish, but she was petrified as it hung lifeless from the hook. I told her it was okay – the fish was dead. I asked her to come over, and as soon as she was close enough, I gave a wee tug on the line and she leaped back with fright.

Given that Hana had the attention of many of the counsellors, I knew I'd have to come up with an original plan to woo her. I decided to tell her future by way of a pack of playing cards. Of course, I had no idea what I was doing, but if I pulled it off with dexterity and guile, I had a chance of success. To ensure I didn't cheat, Hana turned all the cards herself. As she turned the cards, I closed my eyes and told her stories about her future.

Each card was followed with a faux story, all leading to the big reveal. She'd marry in a few years and have two children. She'd live in a big house. The relationship would be a rocky one, but she'd eventually find happiness.

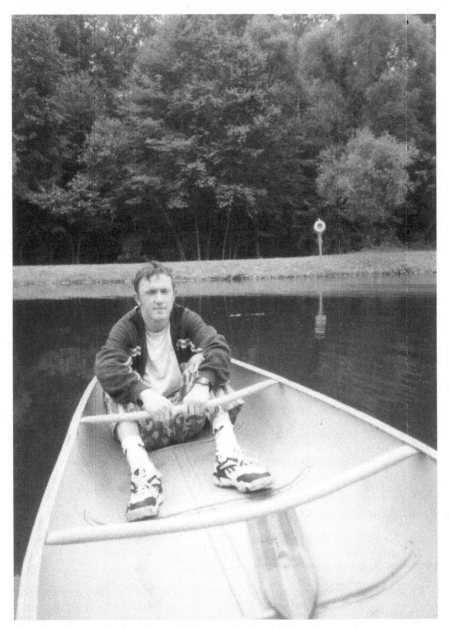

On the lake at Camp Merry Heart – Hana is doing the rowing!

After a few minutes of loss of signal from the nether land – or running out of bullshit – I decided it was time. Once she turned over the six of diamonds, I gasped in mock disbelief. She was suddenly alarmed. I paused for effect, let the silence linger a bit more. It was so secret, I couldn't tell her until everybody had left.

Once we were alone, I beckoned her towards me. I wanted to whisper in her ear. I told her she was a fantastic kisser. She smiled and proved it.

Camp Merry Heart was the total inverse of l'Arche, because it was American. The Yanks strive to do everything bigger and better. Maybe had I stayed for longer in Trosly-Breuil, I would have grown accustomed to the slower pace of life. Who knows? But I did know that *this* suited me, without forcing me to change.

Work. Sleep. Work. Sleep. We had the odd weekend off, and the British and Irish went off drinking, but that never appealed to me. I was content to stay at home on the camp decking and work on my flirting. Someone described it to me as living a whole year in fast-forward. We had Christmas, we had Halloween, we had summer holidays – all four seasons in three months. It was a goldfish bowl, where everybody knew what you were up to. Relationships had to work quickly, because there was so little time. Relationships also broke down quickly, because there were new ones to be made. Nigel was a demigod with all the women. He tried and succeeded, tried and failed, succeeded, succeeded and succeeded.

Graham, a Scottish rugby international, had lots of time for me. Despite being like the President of Camp Merry Heart, he always confided in me. Between him, Nigel, Shane and Jarkko, my confidence was boosted to much higher levels. I was always a cocky wee shit, but I also thrived in the company of better men than me. I learned from them; I castigated them

(Nigel mostly); I was made to feel six feet tall in their company. It was as though Graham was lifting me in one of his lineouts. And they needed me, to be this father figure. I could be that. This responsible head. A massive thing was that they trusted me, as a sort of counsellor to the Gods. They came to me for advice, and I was quite happy to play the civil servant to their political heads. Working away behind the scenes, in the background.

They included me so seamlessly that I couldn't help but compare it to home, to how my schoolmates and ex-team-mates in Navan never did. This new me. This *broken* me. Well, a few, like Kenneth and Padraig and Darren, were there for me, but others walked away, heads down, because they couldn't handle what happened or didn't know what to think. Maybe I'm still disgusting to them?

Nigel, Shane and Graham always treated me well. They joined me for drinks in Navan man Barry McCormack's bar in Manhattan when we

Graham and I at Camp Merry Heart, 1996.

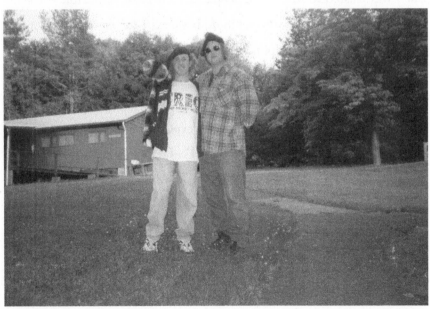

needed time away from the camp, even when I was only on the shandies. Nigel slagged me off. He said I was a 'poofter' for not drinking. I always laughed it off. They included me. Accepted me. I never felt it was put on. They wanted to be in my company. Made me laugh. At times, they took the piss out of my disability. The right way. Laughing with me. Using humour.

But the biggest realisation from Camp Merry Heart didn't kick in until I had been there for about a month. Suddenly it dawned on me that I was now responsible for adults and children with disabilities, the way only a few years ago, people were responsible for me. I was their everything, the way the staff in Beaumont and Dún Laoghaire were once mine. They relied on me to do it all for them, just like I once had. It was a freeing feeling, even when I was designated arse-wiper-in-chief.

Sure, it could be mentally draining to arrive on a snow scene of talcum powder, with the camper eating moisturiser, and having to clean that up. But I was trusted to help these people at their most vulnerable – I knew what that was like, being unable to do basic stuff for myself – and it was empowering. Of course, wiping someone else's arse is unpleasant, but when you remember why you have to do it, and the journey it took to put you in this position, then it's not so bad.

Hana and I continued our romantic explorations for the entire three months, and she accompanied me to the Camp Oscars on our last night at Merry Heart. I'd had a brainwave that we should attend the event in tuxedos, and even managed to blag a discount on their rental when I told the lady in the shop that myself, Nigel and Graham were attending the World Rugby Awards. To nobody's surprise, Nigel won Camp Casanova, but I was delighted to take away Best Camp Rapport.

When it came to saying goodbye to Hackettstown, Hana had initially planned to travel in the opposite direction to me. However, as we got closer to departure, she changed her mind and we made our way to New York. From there it was on to Pittsburgh, Chicago, Omaha, Denver, Phoenix, Vegas and LA. The boy who struggled to walk a few steps just a couple of years ago sure was getting around.

Dressed to the nines for the Camp Merry Heart end of season party (I'm on the right).

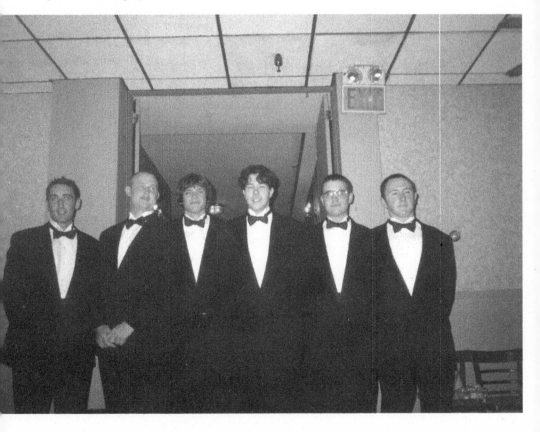

CHAPTER 9

I WAS JUST CHANCING MY ARM

7 JANUARY 2021 – THIRTY-ONE YEARS AFTER THE INJURY

I can't remember what my first impression was when I saw Phil for the first time, but I can remember that he seemed to be kind of different from other guys.

I could not recognise the reason from the beginning; only later, when I got to know him better, I realised that the experience he'd had from his childhood probably had a strong impact on him and his personality. He always seemed to be much more mature than other people of the same age. I could feel patience and some kindness from him whatever he did and whoever he was dealing with.

He always had quite a strong sense of humour, sometimes a little bit sharp … like when he stood at our family doorstep in Brno without letting me know first! I was glad to see him and just about ready to kill him at the same time. I really hate surprises.

Now that I look back, I never looked upon him as a disabled person, I think. Of course, I knew he had some limits when it came to living an ordinary life, but he attracted me with his personality.

When I was with him, I felt that everything had a solution and that he had a reasonable approach to life … that was more important for me I guess.

I can remember one moment, at the end of the summer in New York, in particular. We were walking in Central Park and there were some in-line skaters passing by. I said, 'Oh, I'd like to go skating.' And he just said, 'Not with me.' That was the first time I realised he was actually disabled.

Hana Klimemtova, Phil Quinlan's ex-girlfriend

SEPTEMBER 2000 – ELEVEN YEARS AFTER THE INJURY

The Olympic Stadium in Sydney is far emptier than it should be for a final. Especially considering just a few minutes ago a crowd of 112,524 were crammed in here to see Cathy Freeman romp home in the 400 metres. But I suppose the whole country is probably celebrating her win right now.

And I shouldn't really complain. I'm not actually supposed to be here. Not just because I don't have a ticket. But because my chances of surviving my injury were just twenty-five percent.

I rub my ear and take a breath. I think about the boy from Navan who dreamed for so long of wearing the green singlet of Ireland in an Olympic final and look down at the crippled leg of the man who instead wobbled his way past security and hid in a toilet to watch another Irish athlete go for gold.

It was Jack Finn, my GP, who convinced me to travel Down Under in 1999, because he was coming here with the Irish International Rules side as the team doctor. He knew I'd been bitten by the travel bug, that I wanted to put some distance between myself and all that I can't leave behind. He suggested that I approach the *Meath Chronicle* to offer my services. While I didn't have any discernible qualifications for the role, other than the fact that I liked sports and I'd reported on the school's GAA matches for Kevin Mallon, they were only delighted to have boots on the ground for the series.

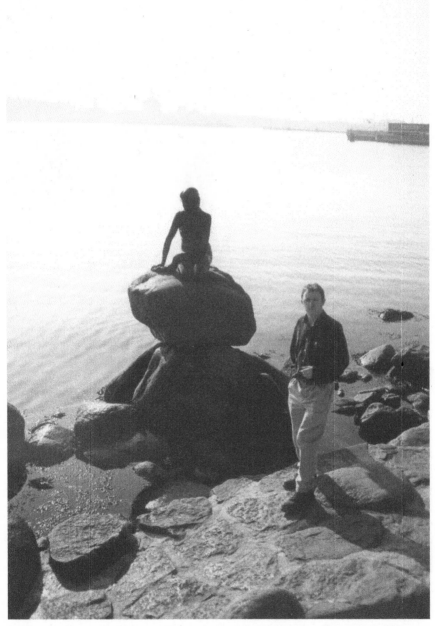

Bitten by the travel bug: In Copenhagen, en route to a Finnish wedding, 1999.

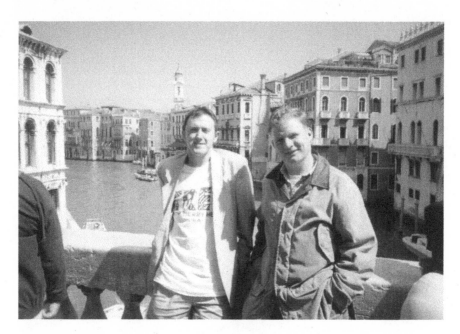

Myself and Shane exploring Venice.

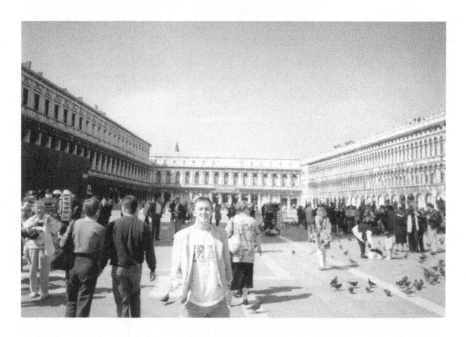

I spent a few days getting my vaccinations, preparing for the off, and gathering names and addresses of contacts I'd need couches or floors from. Mam and Dad dropped me to the airport early one morning. As we said our goodbyes, it was hard to read their faces. They'd wrapped me in cotton wool for the past few years and now here I was, disabled, flying about as far away from Navan as you can possibly go.

I arrived in Melbourne on a one-way ticket and with £300 in my arse pocket. My plan, back-of-a-stamp as it might have been, was to work the International Rules series, then stick around another year for the Olympics.

When I got to Melbourne, Frank Roche of the *Evening Herald* helped me get my accreditation straight away. I hardly needed it, however, as when I met the team, I was just another one of the Meath lads. Colm O'Rourke and Trevor Giles knew me from school, while Darren Fay, Graham Geraghty, John McDermott and Mocky Regan were happy to hear another familiar accent. I even met the great Jim Stynes in the toilets of the great MCG stadium, at the after party. He seemed very interested in my story, until he was pulled away to meet someone more important. A gentleman though.

I covered the series as best as I could, even if overzealous security tried to bar me from the press box for the opening game at the MCG for not wearing a shirt and tie.

Before I even arrived in Australia, I knew sports journalism wouldn't sustain me for the whole year up to the Olympics – even if Michael O'Muircheartaigh was working in the seat next to me. What use would the *Meath Chronicle* have for coverage of Aussie rules or rugby league? So I had sent my CV to a few recruitment agencies before leaving home. They still wanted to meet me face to face, just to make sure I was real and to test me on my computer skills.

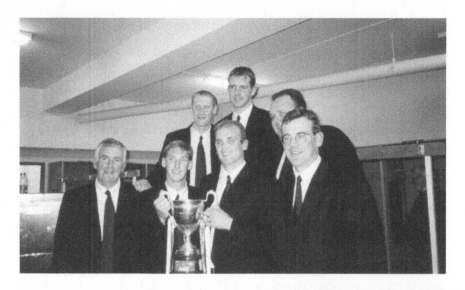

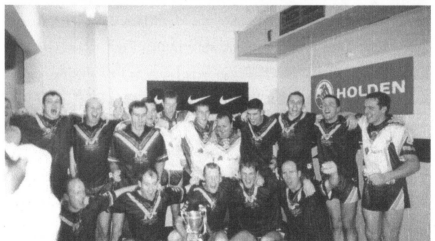

The Meathmen in 1999 after the International Rules test win against the Aussies.

My VISA meant that I could only work for any one company for a maximum of three months at a time. To be honest, that was perfect, because I really didn't want to spend too much time in one spot. I might not be able to move fast, but that doesn't mean I wanted to stay still for long.

Travelling throughout Australia was a huge release. Like on my other adventures, fellow travellers loved a solitary traveller, even more so one with a limp.

On Kings Canyon. I stumbled up the steps, but came down on my bum.

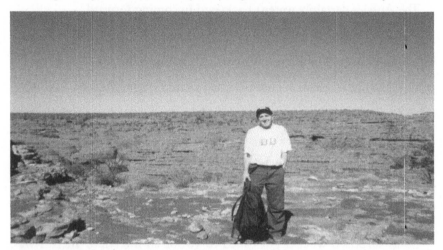

Bondi Beach.

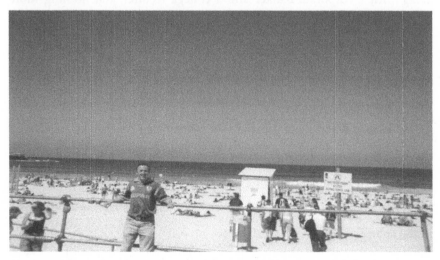

Once, walking into a bar in Alice Springs, I spotted an old cowboy at the bar eyeing me up. As I slowly limped closer, he asked, 'What 'appined ye lig?'

'Oh, I got injured playing football.'

'Aussie rules or rugby league?'

'Soccer!'

'Serves you faaackin' right. What ya drinkin'?'

The Aussies certainly weren't backward in coming forward.

Sydney felt like some sort of spiritual home. So much so that I nearly blessed myself each time I saw the Sydney Opera House, while crossing the bridge, just like a chapel at home. So, as I moved around Australia, working in all sorts of temporary jobs, I knew the big one I wanted was in Sydney, to work at the Olympics. I had answered an ad in the *Sydney Morning Herald*, but wasn't holding out much hope. Surely, I thought, the locals would snap up all the paid jobs. If I could afford it, I'd have happily worked as a volunteer. The Games meant that much to me.

I was surprised when I got called to go for an interview. There I was, along with a corporate banker and a college lecturer, and nothing more than a cover letter stating that I was the disability officer for St Patrick's Athletic Football Club in Dublin.

The interview itself seemed too easy. I couldn't figure out if they were taking it handy on me because I was disabled or because I was a thick Paddy.

'What would you do if you found a suitcase or a suspicious package at the Games and nobody is attaching themselves to it?'

'I'd clear the area calmly while calling security to deal with it.'

'What would you do if you came across a drunk person causing havoc in the arena?'

'I'd clear the area calmly while calling security to deal with it.'

It really wasn't rocket science.

I was in Darwin when my Sydney housemate, Ciaran, called. There was a letter waiting for me, he said, with the Olympic logo emblazoned on the envelope. I opened it as soon as I got home. I was devastated to read that I had not been selected as a team leader at the Sydney Olympics. But delighted to read that they were offering me an even better position, as manager. I would have danced if my leg had let me.

In my Sydney Olympics uniform, with the stadium in the background.

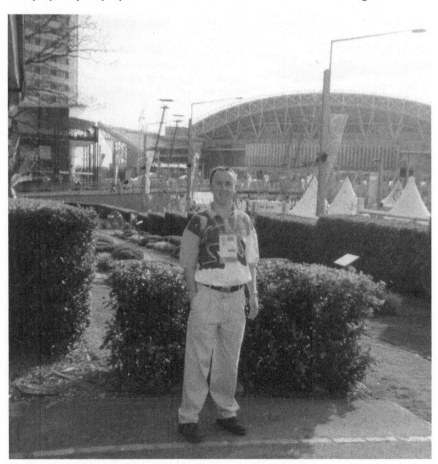

The training was boring, but thankfully brief, and we were given an extensive guided tour of the Olympic Park as part of it. They tricked us too, to keep us on our toes. One morning, the entire train system, and therefore the whole park, ground to a halt. I had to work an eighteen-hour shift that day and slept on a sofa in one of the meeting rooms. Word came through the next day that this was just a test to put us through our paces, and we'd passed.

The Games themselves started on 15 September, but I had to be on site for a couple of weeks in the leadup to the opening ceremony. As I walked up to Central Operations, my superior, who I'd never met before, asked me what had happened to my leg. 'Shite,' I thought to myself. I didn't go into too many details, as I just didn't need to have the conversation just then. I told her it was a sports injury and that seemed to appease her.

Central Operations could be found between Herb Elliot Avenue and Dawn Fraser Avenue, sandwiched between Showground Road and the Olympic Park Convenience Store. No matter how many times I visited the building, I always had to pinch myself: I was at the Olympic Games!

Due to the nature of my role, I didn't have free access to any of the events, but we could get special tickets. The three events I had on my list were Terry McHugh in the javelin; the men's 4X100-metre final; and a golden ticket to see Sonia in the 5000-metre final. I knew from the get-go that this last would be a challenge, because of Cathy Freeman's race just before.

Terry McHugh's event was much easier to score tickets for, but when I got inside, he was throwing from the far end of the stadium. All I could see was a pea-sized body and his spear landing close to me.

At one stage, I got up to do some stretching for my back and hamstrings, and was tapped on the shoulder by an elderly volunteer. He saw my Irish

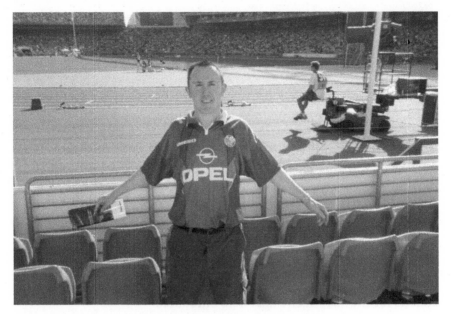

In the athletes' enclosure at the 2000 Olympic Games.

football jersey, with 'Quinlan' on the back, and he presumed I was an athlete. He said that I should really do my stretches in the athletes' enclosure, because the customers' seats were beginning to fill up.

I waited for Terry to return to the enclosure and shook his hand, commiserating with him.

'Phil Quinlan?' he said when I introduced myself by my first name.

'Yeah, that's me,' I replied, stunned.

He told me that his mother – who lived close to mine in Silverlawn – had said that I would be at the Games and to keep an eye out for me.

And that's how I got to tonight. The night Sonia O'Sullivan would surely see the tricolour raised high into the Sydney sky. As expected, I hadn't managed to secure a ticket. Even though I was off work, I chanced my arm and arrived in my full uniform, complete with accreditation, to try to get some of the atmosphere.

The first place I wobbled to was the side of the stadium where I knew I might have a better chance of getting in. It was still going to be tough. Everyone was expecting Freeman to win, so security was tight. A bloke that had trained with me spotted me and tried to usher me in as a guest, but his superior gave him a bollocking.

Dejected, I was tempted to shuffle as fast as I could back to Central Ops to watch Sonia's final on the telly. But then, miraculously, the stadium started to empty. Cathy Freeman's fans had gotten the result they wanted and were leaving in their droves. Security was so focused on those exiting that I had a chance to swim against the tide of human celebration. It worked, but the stadium was still quite full, so I hid in a bathroom until the athletes for the 5000-metre final were introduced.

When I heard Sonia's name announced, I made my way up the steps into the stadium. Sonia was in the form of her life. A season's best in both the heats and the semi-final. I could only imagine what the coverage was like back home; a nation holding its breath on the biggest stage for the second time in a decade.

The race was run at a decent clip. But with 1000 metres to go, Sonia was boxed in and her Romanian nemesis, Gabriela Szabo, was controlling the tempo. I was doing everything I could in the stands to run the race for her. Roaring at her to get onto Szabo's shoulder.

When the bell went, she did just that, and made her way into second place. But the little Romanian responded.

I had been watching most of the race with one eye on security, but now I couldn't take my eyes off the track. 150 metres to go. Sonia makes her move. I scream at the track: 'Come on, Sonia!' Everyone left is suddenly Irish, like the Olympic Stadium has by sheer force of will been transported to Cobh.

100 metres to go. This is it. The patented O'Sullivan kick.

I'm on my feet, willing her over the line with every fibre of my being.

She's going to do it.

She's going to pass her.

But she doesn't.

Second. A silver medal.

I slump into my seat. Dejected.

The stadium is almost silent. Sonia is stunned.

It's only now, devastated by her defeat, that I realise this wasn't only Sonia's race. This was *my* race too. This was everything I'd ever wanted as a kid. From running in the streets of Kitwe to the fields of Navan.

And as Sonia's heart broke, so did mine. She'd have more events to compete in, more medals to win. But my race was run. I was always going to be disabled. A runner-up forever.

CHAPTER 10

AND WE'LL PAINT BY NUMBERS

25 DECEMBER 1989 – ONE MONTH AFTER THE INJURY

I was sitting on Neil and Dee's sitting room floor in Trim, visiting with Mam and Dad. I don't think we were there that long. Neil & Dee had two phones in the house, in the hall and kitchen.

I think Dee was in the kitchen when the phone started to ring. Confused and worried, she handed the phone to Mam. It was said Philip injured himself playing a match and we had to go back to Navan to make sure he was okay. Mam and Dad said to us that you'd be grand as we drove back in the car. I believed them. But looking back on it now, it was how they sheltered or protected us from the real truth.

'Phil has to go to Dublin because there are better doctors there. He'll be home in no time.'

I remember visiting Beaumont Hospital all the time, but not being allowed into the intensive care unit. Only adults were allowed in. I remember asking all the time could I go in and see you, and eventually Mam said yes. As we walked in, I was okay until I saw you laying there hooked up to big machines and endless tubes. My job was to tell you to breathe when you forgot to and the big machine would beep!

That's when it hit me and I just burst out crying. I will never forget that.

But as always, Mam, Dad, Nanny and Francie would say that you were
just having a rest and you would be okay.

I'm not sure when exactly this was, but I was earwigging when doctors
were talking to Mam and I knew something wasn't right. There were chairs
just outside the intensive care unit. I remember peeping my head around
the corner, looking down the hallway and seeing Mam on her own with her
head in her hands, crying.

This was the first time it crossed my mind that I might grow up without a
big brother.

James Quinlan, Phil's brother

2006 – SEVENTEEN YEARS AFTER THE INJURY

I've always had an interest in working in education, but never thought it
would amount to much. I had completed two special needs assistant (SNA)
courses with the Midland College of Childcare, paying quite substantially
for both courses. I loved being able to type up all assignments, and often
offered my typing services to the older ladies who hadn't access to a computer.

Even when I was studying and flying through the courses, it was only
ever a hobby. A hobby that I really enjoyed. I very much enjoyed my week's
work experience in St Anne's Special Needs School on the Curragh. But I
parked the idea of ever becoming an SNA.

However, in 2006, I approached Patricia Fahy, a friend and principal
of St Paul's School at the time. She said that I should chance my arm
with St Mary's Special School in Johnstown, Navan. The principal really
enjoyed listening to my story, my experience at working in l'Arche and,
more importantly, being a counsellor at Camp Merry Heart, which I knew

would stand to me. I was schooled for the interview and then I got called shortly afterwards saying I was being offered a job.

Handing in my two months' notice at Modus, I was relieved to be leaving the bad atmosphere. I was dropping €10,000 in salary but, after doing my due diligence, I knew I could move back to Navan, live on the breadline for a year or two, and then, as the years progressed, my wages would go up.

What I hadn't prepared for was how hard it would be physically. Sitting on my bum for eight- to ten-hour days in Modus hadn't done my body much good. I learned very quickly on the first day, when I was told to sit beside two bulky teenage boys. As they learned to trust me, we'd go on to be great friends.

Doing buses became impossible for me, because of the physical nature of having to traverse the length of a football pitch, on terrible surfaces and gradients, writing down what order the buses would be in to collect the kids. I was given different, computer-based work, which nobody wanted to do but, in all honesty, suited me perfectly. I scanned photos for the kids, helped them work on the computers, compiled presentations for the school leavers and set up the first school website with the help of a couple of students, which I enjoyed immensely. Working with the children was easy, as they trusted me, but accompanying them out into the schoolyard was quite dangerous. A wide-open space for me is never good. There's nothing to fall against when the legs gave way, a regular occurrence. Not much to lean against for assurance.

Eventually sense was seen and I was posted to a new classroom in the special care unit, away from the main school. This was a Godsend, because all the floors in the building were proper concrete-covered laminate surfaces and everything was inside. In the main school, the bounciness of the prefab floors often set me off balance. Thankfully I only ever came crashing down a couple of times.

The special care unit was inspirational. The kids here were full of personality and I enjoyed having the chats with them and working alongside them. Despite their not being able to walk, talk or sometimes even eat, I always felt pulled towards them. My aim was to make them smile and ensure they were comfortable, safe and happy.

The physical aspect had been reduced to pushing the children in their wheelchairs or heavier, more awkward pods, but I could do this. I could use them as my zimmer frame, which was much safer all around.

The fact that this is, in reality, largely palliative care means the loss of children regularly enough. It was a bloody killer when the first few kids died over my first years there. The bond I'd built up with the wee ones was immense. You're there to work with them, to play with them; you're inches from them, trying to make them smile, hoping to make them laugh. The deep belly laughs that the kids would produce from some simple thing I did made me cry. Pretending to fall about the classroom, sometimes not pretending and honestly injuring myself with a nasty bruise or a sprained wrist from catching myself on the floor. The pain would always be forgotten as they would almost fall out of their wheelchairs or high-lo chairs with laughter. This is why I love the job. This is what makes my day. Making their day.

The palliative care aspect is hard. Palliative care needs a certain personality, and especially palliative care for children. When they're sick or ailing, we're sometimes the first to notice because we're spending hours a day face to face. A slight change in health is sometimes hard to notice, but my gut is normally right.

Trying to get them to communicate is an obvious target. I was working with one wee girl for about five years, with the Speech and Language Therapists (SLTs) giving me all the tools and training to target these skills. However, despite all our combined efforts, we were all at a loss.

One afternoon, I was doing TACPAC (Touch and Communication Package) with this kid. This is a sensory programme in which various different materials are used along to quiet music. Nice and calmly.

1. Using a fan to gently fan their face and body
2. Tapping with a spatula all over the body
3. Flicking with little mops
4. Tapping with pot scours
5. Kneading with hands
6. Relaxation

Because it was a Friday afternoon and we'd come back from a short walk around the grounds with the children, I was particularly tired. I went through the first two steps but on step three, flicking with little mops, I just stopped for a brief second. Being lazy.

Suddenly, the little girl's hand reached out for mine to keep going. I was flabbergasted. I went on flicking the little mop against her arm for another few seconds, and this time stopped on purpose. She grabbed my hand again. Revelation. I kept going, stopping, she'd grab me and I'd start again! I was giddy with excitement and couldn't wait to tell the SLT when I saw her next.

Once the SLT saw what I'd found, she immediately tried it herself, because it couldn't just be me. She was almost crying with delight that after all these years, the child was now wilfully requesting something.

It is very intense, observing the kids and trying to implement something that takes months, if not years. I'd mimic their vocalisations and record it on a Big Mac device, a technique called intensive interaction. The child would then press the Big Mac, hear their vocals in my dulcet tones, and burst out laughing. Like they were telling themselves a very funny joke.

When these kids smile or laugh, it melts my heart. This is a huge reason I enjoy working with them so much.

So you can see why losing these kids is terribly sad. We invest so much in them, and we become like an extra limb for them. A voice. A way of communicating. There was one child in particular, whose grandparents I grew up with and whose parents I knew quite well. Lovely people. I was designated as this child's key worker by the teacher, because she had become quite anxious and it was deemed that she'd need me as the constant in her school life. I rarely missed work. I was part of the furniture. Never sick, despite my disability.

This assignment suited me fine. I could cater for this girl very well. It was so obvious how much her family loved her, doting on her despite her huge physical and intellectual disabilities. Her parents always had a word for me whenever collecting or dropping her off to the special care unit. She was the youngest ever competitor to compete the Dublin marathon, being pushed by her father around the course in her specially made buggy.

She seemed to be her usual self on a certain day in December, and we had a great laugh entertaining her and making her laugh as usual. But the next morning, when she didn't arrive at school, I was told that she had died. I was gutted. She had been a constant in the class for years and I always looked forward to seeing her arrive. She had a rare personality that she gained from her family.

Whatever about the loss I feel when this happens, there must be a huge void left for the parents. It must be horribly hard to come to terms with losing a child. I know it was hard enough for me to process a child dying, but I've since promised myself I'd be more resilient. It is a job with inevitable consequences. Kids will die. I've chosen to work with them, to ensure they're happy, cared for and tended to. I've promised myself I'll not get so invested in the children in future.

However, I find it impossible to take a step back, to disassociate myself or to harden myself for the inevitable. I always say the next child dying will not make me feel so distraught, but it's one thing telling yourself you've steeled yourself enough. It's another thing when the child actually dies.

But this is why I've stuck with this job for so long. It's the biggest privilege, to be given the responsibility for these children by their parents every day, especially when their time is so short. It's not something that everyone can do, working with kids with such severe and profound disabilities. Some people find it hard to even look at these kids. But maybe I can do it because I know that feeling of being shunned, of hearing parents tell their kids, 'Don't stare,' before hurrying away to save themselves from the embarrassment.

CHAPTER 11

TRUE COLOURS

1 MARCH 2020 – THIRTY-ONE YEARS AFTER THE INJURY

The minibus was lively with small talk, talk of where people were meeting up for going out later, and commands to Kerr Reilly to 'let me out up here' as we drove up the Boreen keel close to Navan hospital.

Suddenly, Kerr snapped like we had never known before. 'I don't suppose any of you are planning on going in to visit Philip? He is in there fighting for his fucking life right now.'

You could hear a pin drop as the sense of shame engulfed us from head to toe as we drove close to the hospital.

Whenever I think of what happened to Philip that day, this is always the starting point. I guess we were too young, too carefree, too self-absorbed to truly appreciate what was happening.

No more than an hour earlier, I had watched from the sidelines as Philip rose for a headed challenge with Ray as Parkvilla and Torro played out a cup match. I was injured, but I remember watching the game closely in my civvies from the dugout along with the subs and a few other spectators, including Stephen 'Bisto' Murray.

'Crack' – the sound of the clash of heads was audible, even though it was not the worst coming together of heads that you might see.

Philip duly got attention and was taken off, not feeling the best. Nothing too serious though. Nothing to get overly worried about.

It was not long before someone in the dugout was prodding: 'Philip, wake up Philip.' 'Leave him alone, let him sleep,' Bisto said in his innocence, joking. I don't think any of us knew much more than it was not a good thing to fall asleep after a head injury.

Things quickly became very serious, as it was brought to the attention of the adults present with the emergency services called. I don't remember anything after that point until the jolt in the minibus.

Even if we were not fully aware of it at the time, a small part of all of us died that day. No one knew that more than Philip and his family. I, like others, had the fallback of burying things in the back of my mind, listening for updates on Philip's progress, watching as Philip emerged to walk again, talk again, return slowly but surely to a 'normal' life.

Just like the day it happened, I was able to watch from the sidelines as Philip rose to the challenge, this time supported by a real team.

Damien Hilliard, Phil's Parkvilla teammate

SUMMER 2006 – SEVENTEEN YEARS AFTER THE INJURY

Some of my injuries are obvious. People can see the limp. They know something has happened to me. Some aren't so obvious, and I don't just mean the mental side of things. From the night of the Liverpool v Newcastle match in 2001, when my back went and I had to spend a week in bed, it was never right.

Sometimes I worried that I was just a natural patient. Did I like the attention? Dad always slagged me, saying that I got injured on purpose to avoid sitting the Inter Cert the following summer to watch Italia '90. As excuses go, being in a coma is right up there.

But the truth was, by the start of 2003, I was sick to my back teeth of doctors. The pain in my back and hip was still immense, and only slightly eased by taking Difene. This was the only painkiller that helped dull the stabbing pain. I'd tried valium in an attempt to relax my tense muscles, as directed by the professionals, but ended up firing them into the bin.

I never turned to alcohol; I looked drunk enough as it was. But I tried a cacophony of painkillers and a kaleidoscope of anti-inflammatories before I succumbed to the fact that Difene was my only man. Although it only gave me a minimal amount of relief, I needed this tiny bit of help. Fuck the repercussions; it didn't seem to have much effect on my stomach, so I soldiered on.

The four years after my back injury were a blur of hospital appointments, physio check-ups and pain. The biggest problem was that once a medic took a look at me, they assumed the issue was my awkward gait and didn't think I was worth more exploration. Most didn't even ask. If they did, right then, I'd have described it as walking barefoot on broken glass.

But the way I walked wasn't what caused me problems as I wobbled around the world. Now I couldn't comfortably walk to the shop to pick up the *Sunday Independent*, never mind work the Olympic Games and fill the pages of my passport with visa stamps. In the end, I resorted to Dr Google, because it was a lot less painful to sit down and read on-screen than it was to struggle around to various medical appointments only to be told, 'I'm afraid it's just because of the way you walk, Mr Quinlan.'

It had gotten to the stage where even sitting down was painful. The impact always felt like it knocked something out of whack. If only that could be fixed, I thought, as I searched endless websites – both reputable and not-so-reputable – then I could concentrate on treating my spasticity and tone.

The treatments continued to come and continued to fail. I was treated with nerve root blockers, epidurals, painkillers, muscle relaxants, and was even prescribed a new carbon-fibre AFO (splint), but nothing stopped the pain. I told these orthopaedic surgeons exactly where I thought the pain stemmed from, pointing to my sacroiliac joint and my piriformis, but they didn't want to listen. How could this disabled young man know exactly what was wrong with him? He had never attended medical college!

I enquired about chiropractors, but was told to stay away.

It helped, and probably didn't help, that I was sitting at a desk for eight hours a day, unable to move unless I really needed the toilet. On some days, I just held it in. All day. Colleagues wondered why I didn't take breaks in the canteen, but the massive effort and pain involved in clambering down the mountain of stairs kept me at my desk. Every journey, no matter how insignificant an able-bodied person might think it was, was a nightmare for me. Even thinking about it scared me.

There was an elevator. And unusually, it always worked. But it was at the far side of the building, which meant travelling to and from it doubled my journey. Hardly a convenience.

I didn't want to embarrass myself in front of my colleagues either. One time, when walking past the smoking section on my way home, I was trying to guard my mouth from second-hand smoke. This sudden change in gait meant my right leg suddenly went stiff and I collapsed onto the floor. My colleagues rushed to my aid, but it's much easier for me to get back onto my feet myself, because of the dead weight I become. They were trying to pull me up but ended up hurting me even more.

I knew some of them thought I was being unsociable by not eating with them in the canteen. But I couldn't be arsed telling them why either.

Nobody wants to hear other people complaining. My first boss was very empathetic and remains a friend today, along with some colleagues. However, when she left for pastures new, I was the last man standing. Or falling. So I kept myself to myself.

It was travel that took the most out of me. I'd returned to Parkvilla as club Secretary, which meant travelling by bus from Kildare to Dublin to connect with the Navan bus. I helped organise games against Dermot Keely's Derry City and even Stephen Kenny brought his Bohemians team to Claremont Stadium. I set up the first Parkvilla website. I was serious about this Secretary job.

But the train wasn't really an option. It was too far of a walk from where I lived to the station. Even if I could have managed that, the distance from the train platform in Heuston to where I needed to go may as well have been 1,000 kilometres for all the good it was to me. The walk to the terminal was impossible. Busáras was so much easier.

When I'd get to Navan, I'd be collected by Dad or Pat Quin, the Chairman of the club, and attend the committee meeting. Pat's son Paul, tragically, would die from a head injury sustained on a football pitch a few years later.

There were usually only two or three of us at club meetings, so they didn't last long. Martin Rogers – who, along with Pat, was a Parkvilla legend – was the other omni-present member. An hour or so later, I'd be dropped to the bus stop to return to Busáras, before hopping on the coach back to Kildare Town.

After the sixty-metre walk to my flat and the crawl up the stairs, I'd fall straight into bed. Too tired, too sore, too fucking broken to leave that bed again until morning, I'd leave a Pringles can on the locker beside me to use as a makeshift bedpan. Anything to avoid having to put my back or hip through any more pain.

There was only one thing for it – I was going to have to learn to drive. And once I started, I wished I'd listened to Nigel and started earlier. I thought of him as I followed his parents from Kildare to Newbridge in my little silver three-door Yaris when they were showing me the apartment he wanted me to run.

From that apartment, I could see the rugby pitch on which I thought I'd become the next Tony Ward. But other than that, car or not, life in Newbridge was a lot quieter than Kildare Town had been. But I found joy in driving.

I'd made it my business to visit Nigel's folks once a week. They had always looked after me, so I was damned sure I was going to look after them. I also loved driving aimlessly around the Curragh and learning all about the area.

If only I could go back to the future!

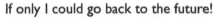

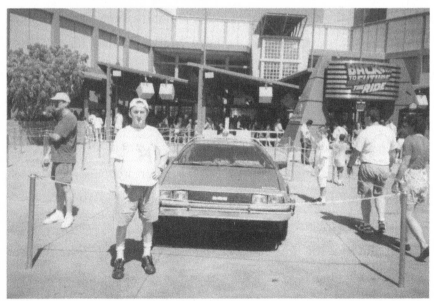

From the Curragh Camp to Donnelly's Hollow, there was always something new to learn. I'd drive to the Curragh racecourse and walk across it. Being softer underfoot than a pavement meant I could stretch out my gait a bit further because the threat of falling and hurting myself was less worrying with the grassy landing.

Sometimes I'd just find a spot on the Curragh and stop and sit, and maybe read a magazine or a newspaper. The odd time it would be something I printed out from the internet about chronic pain. I'd been researching it for years, trying to figure out exactly where the pain was stemming from. Instead of going down for breakfast or lunch at work, I'd stay at my desk trying to find clues and printing out material to digest later.

One day I stumbled across an article which stated that 'chronic pain brings on depression'. I was elated.

Seriously.

I nearly jumped out of my skin. The chronic pain in my back was the reason I'd been feeling very low for the past few years. Just this line alone helped me come to terms with what was going on in my head, more than a therapist could. Not that I was depressed; I had just been feeling terrible, and now I had found out why.

Sometimes I would just drive for hours on end, to nowhere in particular, because I could. I'd pay for it with pain from being seated in the one upright position. But it still gave me freedom, like few other things could.

One thing that definitely helped was swimming. I joined the Keadeen Leisure Centre, where a few lengths of the pool and a sauna would give some relief. The club was full of jockeys who, thankfully, were always happy to talk about things other than horses. This was lucky, as the only steeplechasers I was interested in were Kenyan and running laps of an athletics track.

Outside of driving and the odd swim, I found I kept to myself a lot more in Newbridge than I had in Kildare. I watched a lot of TV and if I was hungry I'd tip into town to the chipper. I'd usually have my dinner at work and something light when I got home. The local chipper also imported Italian wine, which he sold on the side for a fiver a bottle. A lovely Chianti was the star of the show. I was accountable to nobody and could wobble into bed as early or as late as I wanted.

My neighbours in College Orchard were decent and not long after moving in, I started a relationship with the physio upstairs. She was great in every way, but a smoker, which I despised. She lived in the apartment directly above mine and gave me some great advice on the stretches and exercises I should be doing. She even mentioned I should get Botox – to loosen up my very tight hamstrings. Seemingly, there are two different strains of botox – every day's a school day – one for tightening up muscles and the other for loosening them. Once injected, I would undergo a serious stretching regime that would, in theory, lengthen my hamstrings. I was game for anything.

I was two years waiting for an appointment with Ger Hartmann, physiotherapist to the stars. To get to him in Limerick, I had to drive through all the small towns and villages along the way. I called in to see Dad's auld mate, Seamus Darby, in his Greyhound Bar in Toomevara.

I had to park about 100 metres from Hartmann's surgery in Limerick city centre, which provided a great way to warm up for the physio session after the long drive down. When I reached the office, I overheard a conversation between the receptionist and Haile Gebrselassie, whom I'd seen claim gold in the 10,000 metres a few years earlier. He was at the airport and waiting for a lift. I regret not driving out to the airport and ferrying him back into the clinic myself. Once more, I missed out on Olympic gold.

Hartmann hurt me. Fuck, he hurt me. He pulled me apart. He stuck his huge fingers into areas of my body that left me reeling in agony. He dry-needled me, which was a new and painful experience. I'd always had a high pain threshold for the 'macro' things, like trying to walk with severe back pain or knee trouble. I'd got on with it despite the pain. However, needles, I've always felt acutely.

He handed me over to another Ger, his assistant, who took me through some stretching exercises that would help alleviate the pain in my hip/back area.

The second time I went, I met Ronan O'Gara on the physio table. He saluted me and told me that he was trying to avoid surgery, that hopefully Hartmann would have him ready for the upcoming British and Irish Lions Tour to New Zealand. In Ger's hands, he made it onto the plane. For me though, he couldn't do all that much. I was no Ronan O'Gara.

My GP, frustrated with my pains, referred me to Eanna Falvey, Irish rugby team doctor. He shook my hand on arrival, studied me walking into his office, listened to me on the way and within seconds diagnosed not my patellar tendon as the cause of the pain, but referred pain from my weakened calf. He's used to diagnosing rugby players in the heat of action and must determine, within seconds, exactly what's wrong.

He gave me a very simple exercise. Standing with two hands against a wall and stretching out my leg behind me was something I was used to. However, he told me to use a book, place my top two toes on it and stretch again, as normal. The extra stretch hurt the first few times, but my calf eventually eased itself into a stretch I've been doing twice daily since.

The physio living upstairs moved out, replaced by a speech therapist from San Diego. She had hair that, when it caught a certain light, looked ablaze. She had a temper to match too. And I dumped her while watching TV one night, never taking my eyes off the screen. She told me I'd regret it. She told me I'd end up alone. But she was wrong.

In fact, not long afterwards, I even turned down a marriage proposal from another American girl, Katie. I had met Katie years previously in Edinburgh at a crêpe stand in the Grassmarket. I was attending the Scotland v Ireland 5 Nations game and had a spare ticket. I offered, she obliged.

I'd spent a few days with her and her family in California, and she arrived in Newbridge on New Year's Eve the following year. In a restaurant full of punters, she asked me to marry her. The crowd turned immediately to our table in anticipation of my answer, but I was too stunned. I burst out laughing. Seemingly, this is not the reaction any girl wants.

I was on my own again. But I wasn't alone. You're never alone when pain is your constant companion.

JULY 2003 – FOURTEEN YEARS AFTER THE INJURY

Nigel has that twinkle in his eye again, the one he gets when he's up to divilment. I can tell by the way he's pottering around that there's something he wants to tell me, but he hasn't let it slip just yet. But he's building up to it. I know it.

'You'll never guess what, Phil,' he says eventually; barely able to contain the smile waiting to burst onto his face.

'What?'

'I'm after being selected as an escort for the Rose of Tralee,' he says.

'Would you go and shite. You, an escort? Sure they wouldn't let you near those poor girls.'

'Honestly Phil, I have. It's official. I'll be down in Tralee next month, tux and all.'

I'm rarely lost for words, but this time I am. 'I didn't even know you were applying?'

'Ah, I thought, fuck it. It'll be a bit of craic like.'

'You're some man,' I say as I shake my head laughing. Nigel a Rose of Tralee escort. I didn't even realise it until a few minutes ago, but he was born to be a Rose of Tralee escort.

'And even better,' he says, the twinkle in his eye now so bright it was casting a shadow over the Dog Star. You know that girl I'm seeing? The one from work?'

'I do,' I say. 'The one that's not your actual girlfriend?'

He shrugs. He knows I've always been impressed by his success with women. He's never rubbed it in, of course, but he likes to tell his war stories all the same.

'Yeah, she's invited me to her sister's wedding in the City West next month. Between it and the Rose of Tralee, I'll need the car for a good bit. Is that okay?'

I became a lot more reliant on Nigel now because of his car. He never had a problem collecting or driving me home from Kildare to Navan on the weekends. That didn't happen so much recently as I was starting to prefer staying in the flat and wallowing.

But it didn't matter to Nigel, he just loved driving and he'd often bring me to his parents' house in Athgarvan where Teresa, his Mam, would make us all dinner. It wasn't quite as good as my own Mam's cooking, but it hit the spot these days.

'Come on,' he says, knocking me out of my stupor. 'We're going to miss it if you don't hurry up.'

We were on our way to Swifts in Newbridge to watch the opening ceremony of the 2003 Special Olympics. It felt like the whole country was going to be tuning in. I'd actually tried to contact the organisers to see if I could get involved in some capacity. Given my experience at the Olympics in Sydney three years earlier, I thought I was a shoe in. Being disabled hadn't stopped me achieving my ambitions before and, if anything, it was an advantage in this role I thought.

But even after contacting the head office, not only did they not take me on, I hadn't even been called forward for an interview. The opening ceremony was fantastic, full of the best of everything Ireland has to offer. But I couldn't help but wonder, when it was all over, how were Irish people going to behave. I had noticed a shift in behaviour recently. All of a sudden people were talking with me, not to me or at me or around me. They could see me for who I am, and accept that I had a disability without worrying if they might catch it off me.

But I wasn't sure it was permanent. It all felt as fleeting as my balance coming down the stairs.

Swifts is great, one of my favourite spots to be. We'd go out quite a bit in Newbridge, Nigel realised that my lack of interest in returning to Navan these days wasn't a reflection on my parents' company, but that there was something more going on in my head. Because of that, he preferred to have me out socialising with him rather than have me staying at home alone with God knows what sort of thoughts going through my head.

I still didn't like being out too late at night. As much as I enjoyed Swifts it was a battle getting up and down the stairs. I'd sometimes daydream about what would happen if there was a fire or some sort of emergency. I knew I wouldn't make it. The cripple would be crushed on the stairs if I even made it that far.

And that was where my head was at. Catastrophising every situation. I knew the pain was getting to me, but I wasn't quite ready to admit how much it was having an effect. Obviously, my awkward and unstable gait didn't help, but I always felt the orthopaedic surgeons and medics were trying to fix the bigger picture, to somehow cure me of my disability rather than just focusing on the pain and trying to help me get rid of that.

Nigel and I went everywhere together and I loved him for taking such a huge interest in me. He was there that evening in late 2001, when he came over to watch Liverpool take on Newcastle in the Goban Saor pub. Just as I sat down – too quickly or too awkwardly I still don't know –I felt this sudden and agonising pain in my back, just above my hip. I froze instantly, knowing something was seriously wrong. I wasn't a big drinker, but, to the surprise of Tom behind the bar, I decided to have a couple of bottles of beer to hopefully numb the pain a little bit.

Nigel had to leave just before the final whistle, but he knew I didn't have far to walk, even with my hobble. But the pain, after just a few steps, was incredible and I stumbled against the wall. The locals all knew I was a wobbler, and this was normal for them, so no one approached me to see if I was okay. But every swing of my right leg brought more and more pain and I had to struggle up the stairs to my bedroom on all fours to make it into bed. A good night's sleep would have me right for work in the morning, I thought.

And when I woke, it seemed to do the trick. But the second I put my foot on the floor I fell, crashing to the wooden floor in extreme pain. I rang my doctor in Navan, Jack Finn, who said he'd phone the local chemist and somebody could collect painkillers for me.

I stayed a week in bed but eventually had to start going about my business again. Even on the best of days, after walking to and from work in Kildare Town, my muscles would have been all tense and strict, but they usually relaxed once I settled down for the evening. Not so now. The pain was unbearable.

But Nigel was like the big brother I never had. He knew my physical limits and would always drop me as close as possible to where we were going to save me a long walk before parking his car. But he didn't baby me either. He knew independence was good for me. When we'd go to the cinema he'd make me walk up the steps on my own. After the movie was over, he'd stand nonchalantly in the aisle waiting for me to shuffle out from my seat and use his shoulder as support on the way down. Gravity was not my friend and he knew it. At the bottom, when I released my grip, I always thanked him, but he'd just shrug it off with a 'no worries mate' as he walked on.

God, if only I could be as comfortable with my own disability as Nigel was I'd be laughing.

He wasn't perfect, mind. For his 30th birthday he'd told me I could bring a friend, so I asked an old banking colleague who had just returned from a stint working as an NGO in Africa. He'd never met her before but as soon as we walked in he rushed up and said: 'she's not seventeen stone, Phil.' The whole pub could hear it. I was mortified. She was mortified. I never heard from her again.

I tried to bring it up with him once when he was showing me around his newly built apartment a few months after his birthday. Nigel being Nigel he simply shrugged it off.

'So tell me more about this woman from the bank, Nigel,' I asked as he was dropping me home.

'Ah never you mind Phil, sure you'll hear all about it before I go to Kerry. And shouldn't you be driving me home now at this stage?'

He was right, I probably should have been. I started taking driving lessons with Joe Kirwin, an instructor with the Irish Wheelchair Association. I'd actually known Joe for years as he lived in Silverlawn with his family.

Because I couldn't use my right foot to control the accelerator and brake, the left foot accelerator adapted car was ideal for me. I didn't have the coordination to use my right foot and the spasticity would make it a dangerous combination anyway. If I got nervous, my right leg would suddenly seize up and become so rigid that it would be near impossible to move it to the brake. Not ideal. It always takes a few seconds of intense thinking, ironically enough, to relax my right leg. And Joe would always say they were seconds you wouldn't have when driving.

But I became quite used to driving with my left foot and enjoyed the newfound independence it was giving me. After a few lessons, I began to think about getting a car of my own. I'd already done a lot of study on it, and had decided that I'd get a Toyota Yaris.

Nigel had already arranged that I would move into his apartment once I'd got a car and run that for him. Driving had made me so much more independent. No longer was I at the mercy of Nigel, of Dad, or of anyone else. I was now able to offer my services. The car had become my new legs. The freedom this offered me was indescribable.

So he was right. I probably should have been driving him.

'Next time mate,' I said. 'I owe you that at least.'

AUGUST 2003 – FOURTEEN YEARS AFTER THE INJURY

Rose of Tralee organisers were yesterday trying to come to terms with the tragic death of one of the Festival escorts in a horrific road accident.

Nigel O'Neill was recently selected as one of the 26 young men due to accompany the international Roses when they arrive in Tralee for the big annual contest next Friday.

Nigel, 30, from Newbridge in Co Kildare, worked with IIB Bank in Dublin. He was one of two men who died in a three-vehicle crash on the Naas dual carriageway last weekend. The other victim was Mark Berry, 40, from Skerries, Co Dublin.

Festival escort co-ordinator June Carey said Nigel's death had cast a cloud over the start of the festivities. She added: 'We are all in a state of shock.'

Irish Independent, 17 August 2003

With Nigel on the Champs-Elysées, a few years before he was killed on the Naas dual carriageway.

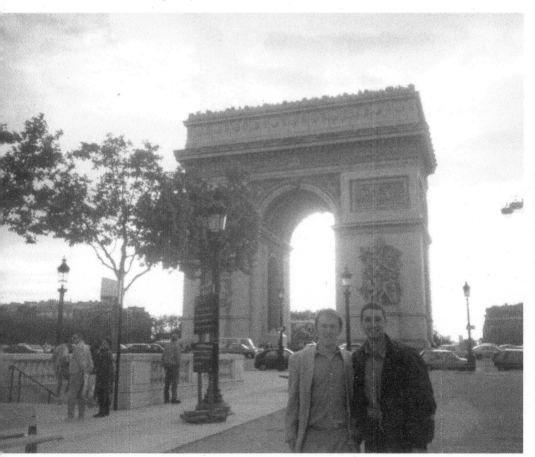

CHAPTER 12

I TOUCHED THE RAINS DOWN IN AFRICA

10 DECEMBER 2022 – THIRTY-THREE YEARS AFTER THE INJURY

From the moment I found myself making mud pies in this wee Irish lad's garden to being shooed out from hiding under his bed by his angry mother when showing solidarity to his mischief, I knew then that Phil and I were kindred spirits.

Though many potato gun adventures were had under the hot African sun, unfortunately and far too prematurely, as with the majority of the mining expatriate community, our paths separated.

We were lost to one other for many years until finally tracking each other down through the wonders of modern technology. I was to learn about Phil's tragic footie incident, his many adventures, and his wish to return to the little sleepy town of Kitwe where our story started so many years before.

Within a blink of an eye, my boyhood friend was on a plane and on his way 'home'. I waited anxiously at our little 'international airport' at Ndola, which was nothing more than the resonance of a colonial, bygone era – a few tin-roof structures that he had last seen as a child.

From the moment I saw this man make his way across the dusty airstrip,
I knew our friendship would endure forever. Finally, when we embraced like
long-lost brothers, it was as if we were instantly kids again, back making
mud pies in his garden.

Karl Hovelmeier, Phil's childhood friend

JULY 2005 – SIXTEEN YEARS AFTER THE INJURY

My first thought on flying into Lusaka Airport was that it looked pretty much the same as it had the last time I'd been in it, some twenty-three years and nine months earlier. Thanks to Ireland's reciprocal visa waiver scheme with Zambia, I could skip the immigration lines and make my way to the VIP section to catch my flight to Ndola, on the Copperbelt.

As I boarded the rickety twelve-seater, I thought of Joey 'The Lips' Fagan in *The Commitments*, who claimed that Buddy Holly's last words were, 'We can't travel in that shit heap.' And if the plane was bad, Ndola International airport beat it, hands down. One runway, and little more than a twenty-square-metre galvanised shed.

But when I saw the huge frame of Karl Hovelmeier, my first ever best friend, waiting to meet me nearly twenty-four years after I had said goodbye to him, I forgot all about my travels and my travails.

'Welcome to Kitwe,' the sign proclaimed as we sped by all the compounds, mud huts and shacks along the roadside. Decrepit blue Hiace public buses trundled by, mostly overcrowded.

When we arrived at Kitana Trust, the school I'd attended as a seven-year-old, the deputy headmaster seemed stunned that we would want a return visit after so long. But he showed us around. Honestly, I didn't really recognise the place at first, but when I spotted the stage area, the brain fog lifted a bit as I remembered my role in *Three Billy Goats Gruff.*

However, it wasn't until we got to 151 Kalungwishi Street that the levees burst and the memories came flooding back. 'Shani Mammy,' Karl said, using local lingo to address a woman who came to meet us at the gate. 'My friend from Europe lived in this house twenty-four years ago.' Soon, we were joined by the rest of the household, who seemed suspicious of my story. That was until I made my way around to the back of the house and pointed upwards in delight, 'I see my mango tree is still here!' That's when they knew I wasn't acting the goat.

My banana trees were gone and the fishpond I'd dug out nearly a quarter of a century earlier was now a stunning flower bed. Karl recalled playing with me, making mud pies underneath the shade of my mango tree. I spotted my old bedroom too. The vegetable patch that adorned the back of the garden and the shed where I tested out my latest concoctions – and tried it on any guinea pig visitors – still stood.

But things had changed too. The house behind us, which seemed so far

151 Kalungwishi Street, with Karl – the first house I remember growing up in.

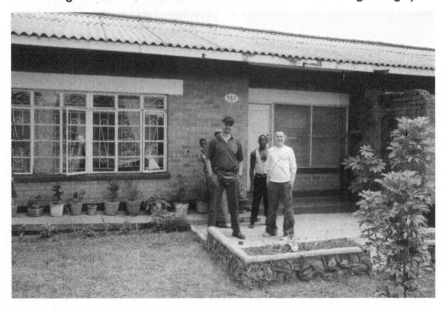

away when I was last here, now felt just a few steps away. Around the front, the copper tap where my sister was electrocuted was gone too, possibly because of said electrocution.

Everything just felt bigger back then. I guess it does when you're seven.

When we got to the Hovelmeier's place – Bok 'n' Rose – I was exhausted. I tried to stretch out the back, but I was in agony.

The next day, we visited the swimming pool at the Italian Club where Keith nearly drowned all those years ago. Again, it seemed impossibly small. Surely he'd have been able to make it to the side himself?

Next on the agenda was Diggers Rugby Club. Oddly enough, this seemed bigger than I remembered. I got a few beers in and we went outside onto the pitch. I didn't remember the grandstand on the right at all. But we walked to the centre of the floodlit pitch with darkness well upon us. I

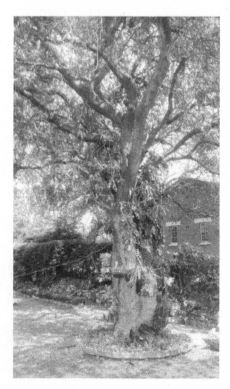

My mango tree, still standing in the yard in Kalungwishi Street! This was my Playstation, my XBox, my Nintendo.

called Dad from the pitch, and he was delighted to hear where I was phoning from. I scored a mock-try with my beer glass on the way back to the clubhouse.

I had vague recollections of the changing rooms and the room where we had the Christmas party with Big Bird in attendance – an appearance that frightened my sister so much she developed a pathological fear of all birds. But some of it was new too. I wasn't allowed into the bar area as a child, but looking at the room all these years later, I recognised a few of the names adorning wooden plaques on the wall: S. Sullivan, B. Mutale, B. Hovelmeier. There aren't many team photos left, as they were all borrowed indefinitely throughout the years.

That was it for Kitwe, and I set off to see the rest of Zambia. It was smaller than I remembered, but my heart was fuller for it.

On top of the usual tourist trinkets I brought home, I also carried a new-found determination to get to the root of my pain. For the most part, it had been okay when I was travelling – the African heat, much like the sauna, played its part in that.

By chance, I stumbled across a chiropractor who was promoting his new business in Newbridge. When I met Todd Redfearn for the first time, I told him where the pain was coming from and, unlike so many others before him, he listened. He had a good feel around my hips and backside and con-curred that he too thought the pain was coming from where I'd said. My SI joint and my piriformis. He told me to book in to see him the following day, which I did, even though top Irish orthopaedic surgeons reckoned chiros were a waste of time.

But I was tired of being passed from pillar to post with no solutions, so I thought, why not?

Walking up the narrow stairs to his treatment room was difficult, but I had found an empty disabled parking spot close by. Once inside, I lay face-down on his treatment table and, in two seconds, he pushed my sacroiliac joint back into place. The relief I felt was immense. He then massaged my piriformis with his elbow. The agony. He told me to relax for a few minutes before getting up. I drank a glass of water and carefully crept down the stairs. The sudden freedom I felt walking back to the car! This relief was unbelievable.

The chronic back pain had gone, after four years of failed treatments. I was petrified that I would put something out of place again, so I didn't sleep a wink that night. How could some of Ireland's top medical professionals have failed me for so long? A swift manipulation. Two seconds. Two fucking seconds was all it took, after years of pain.

I booked in for nine more sessions, out of loyalty, but never needed them. After all this time, the one thing I always knew to be true was the secret. I knew my own body. I listened to it. I could decipher its every whisper and roar. When someone finally paid heed, I was pain-free.

CHAPTER 13

DANCING IN THE DARK WITH YOU BETWEEN MY ARMS

15 SEPTEMBER 2020 – THIRTY YEARS AFTER THE INJURY

I think, in fairness to the referee, the conditions were just about playable on the day. You couldn't see far, but you could see when the game started. It was only as the game went on that conditions became really bad.

I was on my own with the team that day. The challenge itself was innocuous enough – two lads going after a bouncing ball from a standing position. And, as far as I remember, Phil didn't fall on the ground or anything. But in fairness to the referee, he knew something was up, and he stopped the game and went over to see if Phil was all right. The referee did everything right by my book.

I went out onto the pitch and the referee was asking Phil where he was, how many fingers he was holding up. The usual questions. And Phil was able to answer them all, so we all thought he was all right.

The half-time whistle went, and we were having a bit of chat and suddenly someone said, check on Phil. You were in a bad way.

We loaded you onto the bus, and raced you to the hospital. But by then, the conditions were much, much worse. Every time we tried to pass a car to save some time, we just couldn't. It wasn't safe.

When we got to the hospital, I ran to the door and shouted that we had an emergency. As we unloaded Phil out of the bus, he vomited what looked like black tar. I knew that things were bad, but when that happened, I was really worried. They kicked me out of the hospital though, because I'd only be in the way and Phil's mam and dad were on their way.

My own son is playing now. He's seventeen, 6'4" and a big centre-forward. And I think about him going up for headers. You see some awful whacks, but Phil's was so innocuous. It shows that it doesn't matter how it happens I suppose, but where you get the knock.

Gerry Browne, Phil's manager at Parkvilla

SUMMER 1993 – FOUR YEARS AFTER THE INJURY

By the time the Leaving Certificate was in the bag, everyone in Navan was used to 'the Quinlan boy' limping through life. And to a certain extent, my own anger at what had happened four years earlier had subsided a little. Last year, when I looked in the mirror at this new body – this spastic, ugly, shit-under-my-shoe disgusting, wobbly, vacant new body – I'd fly into such a rage I'd think about never leaving my room again.

But when I glanced at myself now, for the most part, I just got on with things. Walking was still a chore though. I still felt like I was walking on two skinny wooden stilts, the left one a full inch shorter than the right one. If that wasn't enough, there was a two-litre water bottle tied to the right stilt and it was being blown by a wind tunnel fan. With all of this, it was almost like trying to walk on a tightrope just to remain upright. The crippling pains in my feet didn't help either, and nor did the cramps in my calves, the niggles in my knees, my scoliosis or the horrendous aches in my hips. But as I said. I got on with it.

I started discovering girls again too. And though I couldn't shake the feeling that some of them only pretended to be interested in me out of sympathy, or because I was the only guy that listened to them, I told myself that I didn't care very much either. It was the good, sneaky, behind-the-bushes kind of attention, not the wrapped-in-cotton-wool kind of attention I'd grown to be annoyed by at home. But it was also the kind of attention that never had much potential. And, when I was being truly honest with myself, I knew that I often felt unworthy of a relationship. What could any woman want from me? What could I give any woman? Of course, this meant that I ended up sabotaging the dalliance to ensure they realised how beneath them I was.

None of them I treated as badly as Nathalie.

Nathalie was French; she had come to Meath to study. It was something we instantly had in common after I'd spent the previous summer in Trosly-Breuil trying to improve my French for the Leaving. That's why I was introduced to her, as I could act as her translator. French to English was one thing, however; French to Navan quite another.

Nathalie was beautiful. She wore LouLou by Cacheral, a scent I'll never forget. But in reality, she was the most mature person I had ever met. Ours was a clash of cultures too. One evening, she asked me if I'd ever heard of Jean-Paul Sartre. She laughed when I enquired which French rugby team he played for. Much later, I'd discover that Sartre believed that we alone are responsible for everything that we really are. And that, by not exploring the myriad possibilities life presents to us, we alone are responsible for restricting our freedom. Though I probably should have guessed that's what she was getting at when she pushed me into an oak tree, told me that actions speak louder than words, and kissed me tenderly.

I was euphoric just being in her company. Friends were jealous. She oozed sophistication in a way that made me feel I should be wearing a tuxedo just to be in her presence. Of course, I was too young or too stupid to realise that I was in love for the first time. But while every moment in her company felt like a year, the months passed in a heartbeat and Nathalie had to return to France.

That didn't stop us from keeping in touch. We shared a few letters, but my parents' phone bill began to grow immensely as we communicated daily. We'd talk about anything. Everything. We spoke about the big stuff – where we would live, when we'd get married, how many kids we'd have, what we'd both work at. We spoke about the small stuff too – how I found walking today, or what TV shows we were both watching. But we never needed a reason to stay on the phone to each other for ages. 'Vous raccrochez!' 'Non, vous raccrochez!'

The following summer, she invited me to her home village in the Alsace region. Her father, being ever so French, gave us one of his many apartments to stay in. We got to practise what we'd spoken about for months previously. But it was still all so surreal. This broken boy from Meath losing his virginity to a French mistress overlooking the Rhine Valley. Afterwards, as Nathalie slept, I read Paul McGrath's first autobiography, *Ooh! Aah! Paul McGrath: The Black Pearl of Inchicore*.

We kept in touch for a long time afterwards, but familiar doubts began to creep back into my mind. I was so messed up and immature that I honestly didn't know what was going on in my own head. My heart was telling me one thing while my brain injury was contradicting it completely. I wanted to watch the remaining games of the 1994 World Cup. I wanted to watch every daily stage of the Tour de France. Not the thirty-minute Channel 4 highlights. The full French five- or six-hour live versions. Nathalie didn't. It was all about me.

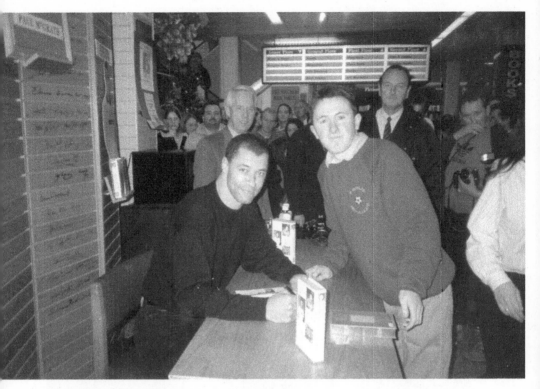

Ooh! Aah! Look who it is!

Daily phone calls became weekly ones. What once seemed like long-ing now felt like clinging. But worse, much worse, niggly feelings of inadequacy became all-consuming doubts. And because I was feeling bad, I hurt her with words – and often lack of words – far more than she ever deserved.

Nathalie returned to Navan one more time. It was 1995, and she was over for my twenty-first birthday party. But by that stage, I was more scared of her than in love with her. Outwardly, I was projecting the image of a macho young man who had overcome a life-changing disability and was far too important for trivial things like girlfriends. But inside, something much darker was taking hold. I was terrified again, like I was when I woke

143

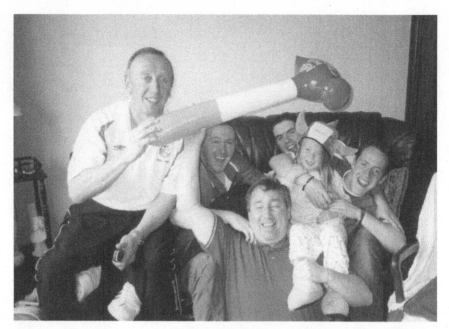

Celebrating Robbie Keane's late equaliser against Germany at the 2002 World Cup.

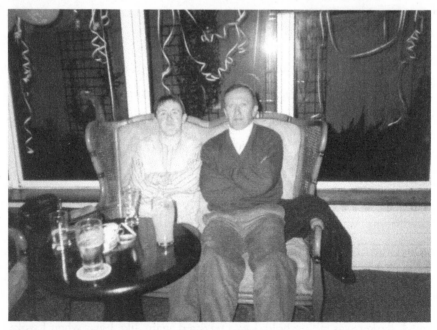

Relaxing with Dad at my twenty-first – still on the rock shandies!

from my coma. I was a battered and bruised little boy suddenly finding himself in a man's body and having absolutely no clue what to do with it.

Every time my inner monologue raised the idea that I hadn't dealt with my injury at all properly, I pushed it deep down, until it converted itself into rage. And despite all my bravado, I was a coward. The night before she was due to fly home, I wrote a letter, trying to explain my thoughts. I failed miserably and knew as soon as I handed it to her. But Nathalie knew. She was always smarter than me. She was always more mature than me. And, in my head, she was always going to be better off without me.

SEPTEMBER 2006 – SEVENTEEN YEARS AFTER THE INJURY

A school has paid tribute to a teacher who died in a collision between a motorcycle and a car in Cumbria.

Nathalie Locicero, of Entry Lane in Kendal, died in hospital following the crash on the A684 between Sedbergh and Kendal near New Hutton.

The 29-year-old was a pillion passenger on the motorbike.

Queen Katherine School in Kendal, where she had worked for six years, described her as a talented language teacher who was much loved.

A statement issued by the school said: 'Staff, students, governors, parents and friends of the Queen Katherine School are in shock at the sudden and untimely death of a much loved teacher.

'Nathalie was a talented languages teacher who had taught at the school for six years. She had energy, enthusiasm and an immense love of life and her chosen profession.

'Her death has touched our community. We miss her very much and send our respects to her family in France and in Ireland.'

BBC News, 28 September 2006

OCTOBER 1998 – NINE YEARS AFTER THE INJURY

I'd been to see Hana in Prague a few times, and each time we'd fall in love a little bit again. This time, the plan was to pay her a surprise visit in her hometown of Brno, and get our relationship sorted out. I was nervous on the train, but my anxiety was calmed by a little girl who sat on her granny's knee across from me. Every time she would glance at me, I would make a funny face and she would burst out laughing. Her granny would then ask what was so funny, as I straightened up my face. The child would point at me and I would pretend to be asleep, leaving the grandmother to scold the child for being so silly.

After traipsing around Brno for hours, and reading a lot of maps, I eventually arrived at Hana's front door. After getting over her initial surprise, she introduced me to Jana, her younger sister, who had lovely eyes and the same unrestrained personality that made me fall in love with Hana in the first place.

Hana brought me up to her bedroom, where I waited a few hours until she had come back from visiting her quadriplegic friend, and Jana prepared a weird noodle and corn salad concoction.

When Hana came home, I was perched sleepily on her bed. I started the ball rolling by asking questions. 'How was your day?' 'What'll we do this evening?' 'Where do you see our relationship going?'

You know, the usual.

We talked for ages and mutually decided to end whatever romantic intentions we had and remain just good friends. A love that had spanned the States, Ireland and the Czech Republic came to an end in a twenty-foot-square bedroom in Brno.

We were due to go to the cinema that evening, one final date. I figured it would be best for me to say goodbye to her parents for the final time then and there. Mrs Klimentova was shaking my hand vigorously as Hana translated her every word at the speed of sound. I offered a few words of thanks, and apologies and goodbyes, to Mrs Klimentova, who smiled lovingly.

Then Mr Klimentova appeared from the living room and offered his hand. He was all smiles, saying something very conspicuous in his native tongue. Hana was doing her best to remedy his words in her translation, but I knew it couldn't be good.

The first time we'd ever met, he had slagged me for the way I looked and the way I walked. I remembered thinking at the time, 'I'll get you back for that, you dick.'

Now I looked him square in the eyes, gave him my most innocent smile, shook his hand and said – in the finest Navan accent, 'Thank you both for your hospitality, your meals and friendly conversation; Oh and by the way, your daughter is great in bed.'

Hana nearly collapsed on the floor with laughter and embarrassment. As she and I left the house for the cinema, the cries of her mother wanting to know what I had just said rang in my ear. At least, that's what I think she was saying.

By the time *Jerry Maguire* was finished and we'd trammed it back to Hana's house, it was nearly 2am. Everyone was asleep. Mrs Klimentova had left me an alarm clock, which I set for the next morning to make sure I would make my train back to Prague.

It duly went off, but when I compared it to my watch, I realised it was fifteen minutes slow. With no time to think, I just grabbed my backpack and ran out the door, racing down the street and taking a sharp left. Racing along the 2km route to the tram station that would take me to the train station, I had a few speed wobbles along the way.

I reached the tram stop just in time to stick out my thumb and halt the bodiless mode of transport. As myself and the driver whirred on into town, I pondered on what might have happened had I gone upstairs to wake Hana.

Tom Cruise might have had Renée Zellweger at hello, but I was never one for big goodbyes. I consoled myself that everything had played out for the best.

CHAPTER 14

I LOVE YOU JUST THE WAY YOU ARE

9 JULY 2020 – THIRTY YEARS AFTER THE INJURY

Unfortunately, we grow up in a society where we are surrounded by judgement on a daily basis. None more so than in a small rural community. Everyone in town knows the drunk, the thief, the adulterer, the teenage pregnant girl and even the 'poor auld cripple'. 'Ah, look at poor Mary there and her poor auld handicapped son Johnny, God love them.' Is it any wonder so many of us grow up with insecurities and inherent bigoted ideas when we are engrossed in such societies from an early age? What many fail to realise is that 'poor auld Johnny' is happy and content with his life and, more often than not, receives unconditional love from Mary that many of us are incapable of understanding.

Having grown up in such a small town, I guess by the time I met Phil I was, unconsciously, quite narrow-minded. Even more so, I was always concerned by judgement or felt judged. But soon after everyone meets Phil, they come to realise that behind every exterior or every stigma there is a real story, a real person, and it's not always our first impressions.

That said, I do remember my very first impression of Phil. I was renting a room in a house he owned; he didn't live in it at the time and all of my dealings with him were over the phone or with his brother. I had never met him in person. What started out as a business relationship somehow managed to make its way into a personal one over emails and text messages. It became pretty clear that we had a mutual love of sport and I always found him very funny in our interactions. So when Phil suggested that we meet up for a date, I thought, 'Sure why not?'

I don't ever recall a conversation about him being injured or disabled, but I think it may have been hinted at or briefly mentioned. On the night of our first date, he had been having dinner with his parents and a few drinks in their house, so I said I'd pick him up from there in a taxi. The taxi pulled up outside his house and out walked Phil – or should I say, out wobbled Phil. Wow, there it was, my first impression: Wow, he's disabled, not just a little limp, but a full-on, partially-paralysed-on-one-side kind of limp.

But I didn't just see Phil. I saw myself and my own judgements too.

Another personal flaw of mine is that I don't like to be different; I want to blend in. But blending in is not something that you can do if you're going out with Phil. I realised that pretty quickly. Initially, I thought every time we walked into a public place, people would look at us and judge us. 'What happened to him? Was he born like that? What's she doing with him?'

But very soon, I moved past this. I saw Phil, not his disability. I now firmly believe so many judgements in society are learned from an early age – nurture over nature. Just as easy as it can be to learn these judgements, I believe they can also be unlearned through education and through visibility. I am so thankful that my kids now grow up in a household where disability is a way of life. It's so heartening to see my kids ask their dad if he needs a hand in from the car, or a shoulder to cross the street. I have no doubt it will shape them into wonderful models of their father.

Helena Quinlan, Phil's wife

SEPTEMBER 2006 – SEVENTEEN YEARS AFTER THE INJURY

I bought a house off the plans at home in Navan along with my baby brother. We decided between us that he would be the one to live in the house and run it for us. It was a no-brainer.

We were always chalk and cheese, but the truth is that I was always incredibly jealous of his popularity, his personality, his ease of partying long into the wee hours and his ability to still play football at a high level. Added to the chronic pains I was experiencing, this put a strain on our relationship at the time. However, he did manage to get some lodgers in pretty quickly.

Because I was living in Newbridge at the time, I rarely had anything to do with the house for the first few months. However, when the first issue with the house cropped up, I was happy to help sort it. One of the tenants phoned to tell me that the boiler had broken down. I had it fixed straight away. The tenant's name was Helena, and she seemed nice, so we stayed in touch. The first time I felt it might be something more than owner-and-tenant communication was when she asked me if I had any plans for the following weekend. I told her I was planning a day of bingeing sport – St Pat's, my old secondary school, were playing in Newbridge; Kildare County were playing in Station Road in the town; and Ireland were playing rugby against England, which I'd watch in Swifts. She replied pretty much straight away that this would be her ideal date.

I didn't act on it then, but eventually the emails became texts and phone calls and I finally plucked up the courage to ask her on a date. I was so excited that she said yes that it was only afterwards I realised I'd picked Mother's Day for our date. Not wanting to disappoint anyone, I arranged to have dinner with Mam and Dad first, and brought Mam a couple of nice bottles of wine. I over-indulged slightly, but all the while I was texting Helena under the table. When she arrived in the taxi, I could see the surprise on her face at my limp. But full of the courage only grapes can bring, I ploughed on with the date. Mam peered out the front window, either to ensure I didn't fall flat on my face, or in an effort to spy on who I was going out with!

In a bizarre twist of fate, front and centre with all his Torro mates at the Royal Meath public house when we arrived was Ray. Him and his mates did their best to 'big me up' in front of Helena, but we were all so drunk I don't think anyone remembered very much the next day.

However, Helena wasn't put off by my disability and soon saw right past it. Quite quickly, our relationship grew serious. Much as I limped around in life, Helena stumbled into my life probably when I needed it most. I knew from Nathalie and all my relationships since that I would end up spending my life with an educated woman. Helena was that and more. She was shy, except when it came to sport. She out-screamed my dad watching 'Match of the Day'. She played football with Oldcastle, winning a county medal with them. And I had more enjoyable chats about football with her than with most of my male mates.

That she knew me so intimately so quickly was incredible. She knows that when I'm in a bad mood, it's invariably to do with my being in pain. I go quiet, I sulk, I feel a certain amount of pride in not showing pain.

Maybe incorrectly. I don't want to encumber her with my worries. I don't ever want to be a burden. That's my greatest fear.

Helena is all too aware of this. After about a year of dating, we stayed a few nights in a particular Wexford hotel, chosen because of its cryotherapy room. This room had a temperature of -110c. It is used to treat injuries in sport.

I've always had a very small portion of hope logged at the back of my mind. A sliver. Just a small sliver. But something that I've always held on to, very deep down. A sort of .001% chance that someday, somehow, through some new-fangled therapy, I'll be healed and back running cross-country for Meath, playing football and rugby and simply able to walk any length without pain. To be able to run again. To be able to run the Dublin marathon. To compete in the Ironman in Hawaii. I'd tried so many therapies, from Botox to nerve blockers, painkilling injections to a large variety of splints. Epidurals, anti-inflammatories and any amount of quacks with mystical cures. There were a couple of trips to Lourdes, harbouring my tiny dreams and those of my parents of some divine intervention. To get me back to what I was pre-injury. Back to the real me. Showing off to Helena in home-made triathlons.

Despite these thousands of failed therapies, I still had a tiny inkling of hope that this cryotherapy was going to help with some of my chronic pains. I was willing to pay the extortionate fee involved for the few minutes of therapy.

We checked into the hotel and I got ready for my treatment. I'd been in touch with the cryotherapy centre before our arrival, and had booked in. When I arrived at their reception, I was handed a simple questionnaire to fill in. Most of the health questions were filled in easily. Any heart conditions? No. Pregnant? Not that I knew of. Severe hypertension, acute or recent myocardial infarction, unstable angina pectoris, arrhythmia, symptomatic cardiovascular disease, cardiac pacemaker? All no.

Ever suffered from blood clots? I had to think about this one. Hard. I did suffer from a blood clot, but only once. That was because of the clash of heads. I was going to write no, but I thought better of it and answered honestly. I wasn't going to take a chance. 'Navan man dies in a cryotherapy clinic because he doesn't disclose that he suffered from blood clots' wasn't a headline I wanted my friends to read. I decided to come clean and state that I did. About twenty years previously, I had had a blood clot. I signed the questionnaire and handed it over to the young guy behind the counter. He left through a side door and was gone for about five minutes. On his return, he had a worried look on his face. He apologised and said that they couldn't let me try it out, because of what I'd disclosed.

I was exasperated and tried to plead my case. It was only once, I said. It hasn't happened since, I said. It was from a clash of heads, I said. I was pleading. Almost on my excruciatingly sore knees.

I'm sorry, he said.

I left the clinic and wobbled towards our room, crying quietly to myself. But I veered into the bar in the hotel instead. This was where real men went to ease their worries. I asked for a pint of Bulmers. I have no idea why. I'd never drank Bulmers. I wanted to get drunk. I wanted to get absolutely sloshed. Piss-faced. Rat-arsed. People see me as a drunk – I'm doing the time, why not commit the crime? Fuck it.

I drank the first pint fairly quickly. I called for a second and was well on my way. Fuck it again. Nobody knew the difference between a sober me and a drunken me. I could pull it off easily. I was always stumbling around the place gripping furniture, like a toddler learning to walk.

Helena, fresh from a relaxing spa treatment, found me not long after my second pint. She gave me a look I knew meant I wouldn't be able to drink a third and helped steady me back to the room. Once inside I cracked. Falling around the room, a phantasmagoria of snot and tears. The bastards, I roared. The tiny bit of hope that I'd be cured of the chronic pains had been dashed. How dare they take that hope from me?

I was inconsolable. Helena tried to stop me from feeling so sorry for myself, which made me cry even more. And I couldn't even get drunk, I shouted. Two pints. Two bloody pints is all I could manage. A cheap fucking drunk. A sorry mess of a man.

I cried myself to sleep that evening and woke up disgusted with my behaviour. I felt guilty for letting Helena down so badly. How she stayed with me after that episode I'll never know, but it changed something in her too. Now she kicks me up the arse when I start feeling sorry for myself, and I love her all the more for it.

I asked Helena to marry me on her birthday. We ate in her favourite restaurant at the time, and I produced the ring. She knew it was coming, but she flapped and fanned her face with New York excitement and said yes. I took to planning our wedding with vigour, and Helena let me. All she had to do was buy her wedding dress and shoes. And lingerie. I organised almost everything else. I haggled with the hotel over extortionate rates. I dealt with all the vendors.

Life was exciting for the two years of the lead-up to the wedding. We were both working and earning, and saving for our wedding. That was it, but it was better than going into debt.

My baby brother James, and best mates Ken and Pádraig, stood beside me and ensured I was in ship-shape.

Father Ray married us in his Oldcastle church, and we had our reception in the Cavan Crystal hotel. Food and service were amazing. Our first wedding dance, ironically, was Billy Joel's, 'I Love You Just the Way You Are!' I overdosed on Difene for the day to take a tiny part of the sting out, but my knees still ached by the end.

We honeymooned in South Africa. By this stage, my right knee had become so bad that I had to use my new wife's shoulder as a crutch. My right leg was in absolute agony for the ten days. I was wheelchaired through the airports but, once out and about, I had to shuffle about everywhere. We chose a wonderfully central accommodation, Waterfront Village in Cape Town, but we still needed to taxi almost everywhere. This was sheer bliss – we had our own deck overlooking the marina; lounging on beds; sipping a cold beer at our own bar. Our very first night was spent at Pigalle, a salubrious restaurant that played jazz and served me the most succulent lobster. It was a long way from Macari's or the Valley in Navan. We were taxied all along the Garden Route, stopping off at serendipitous places along the way.

Helena and I on our wedding day.

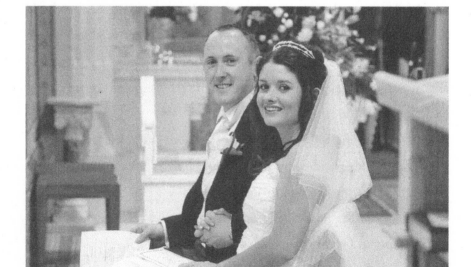

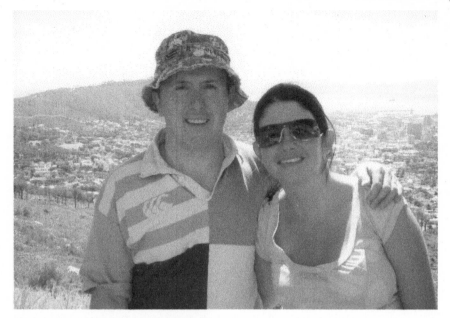

On our honeymoon in South Africa.

It's hard for me to put into words what Helena means to me. Which is a little awkward when I'm writing a book. You hear the expression 'unconditional love' a lot, even though so many relationships are built on conditions. But there is unconditional love between us. She loves me despite having every reason not to. She has saved me from myself more than once. When I'm with her, she doesn't ask me to forget my pain, but rather asks me not to forget who I am, pain and all.

She is everything. And more.

CHAPTER 15

I WAS ONCE LIKE
YOU ARE NOW

2 JUNE 2021 – THIRTY-ONE YEARS AFTER THE INJURY

What's your favourite thing about your dad, Eileen?

'My favourite thing about Dad is that he's funny and smart,' says Eileen.

'Well, my favourite thing is when we both come downstairs early in the morning when you and Mam are still in bed to chat,' Joe counters. 'That and when we go to soccer together.'

What's your favourite thing to do with your dad?

'I like it when we have dinner in Zucchini's, but my absolute favourite time with him was when we went to Harry Potter and went around London for the day,' says Eileen.

'Mine was when we went to France and had lots of fun,' Joe says.

What one thing would you change about your dad?

'I'd like his leg to get better so we can play football,' says Eileen.

'I'd like his leg to get better so we can play football,' says Joe.

Phil's kids Eileen (ten) and Joe (seven)

MAY 2013 – TWENTY-FOUR YEARS AFTER THE INJURY

Helena and myself bought a dog before we got married. Maybe subconsciously we were both preparing for life as parents. A ruby Cavalier King Charles, Helena named him Gooch, after the Kerry footballer. I would train him; Helena would walk him. Any kids we'd have would have to get used to a life with dogs, and also with me doing the talking to them and Helena doing the walking.

I was thirty-six, and in immense pain with my hips, knees and feet, when I learned that we were having a baby. I was ecstatic initially. I was going to be a father. More than that, I was going to be a Dad. My own little bundle of joy to love. Of course, I would love my child unconditionally. But then I began overthinking again …

First-time expectant fathers are naturally bricking it. Having a baby is one of the most momentous parts of a man's life. Things, I was told, would change incredibly. You believe all the horror stories. There'd be no more just leaving the house whenever it suited. There'd be no more late nights getting drunk and lying on the next morning. There'd be no more just doing what I wanted.

Luckily, I was always happy to relax in my house. I was never a big drinker, nor a ravenous socialiser. I'd rarely be in a pub. What was going to change there? I was a homebird now, with a car to get me where I wanted.

Emotionally, though, I wasn't sure I was ready to become a father. Is any man? Emotionally and physically. How would I cope? How could I cope? But of course, there was absolutely no choice. I had to steel myself, upskill myself, cop on to myself.

I'd had it hard over the past decade with chronic pain. I was selfish with my innermost thoughts; I was selfish with my time; I had only just learned to let

Helena into my mind, into my thought processes. Before her, I was better than a priest at keeping secrets. My mind was the confessional. I was a lot more guarded with my thoughts. I never let anybody in. Helena was different.

I was prone to bouts of self-pity whenever anything went wrong for me or when someone close to me made a disparaging remark, slagged me off, tried to get a rise out of me. They always did. It would take me years to overcome being easily risen. Why do those you love the most hurt you the most? I'd have to put all this aside when the baby came along. This baby meant everything to me.

Physically though, that bit was going to be a lot harder. How could I carry a child when I needed every ounce of my being to concentrate just on barely staying upright? I'd been learning to lengthen my stride again after chronic back pain from 2001. Because I'd started driving, there wasn't as much need for me to walk further and recondition my body back to what it was pre-2001, when I was wobbling around the world, awkwardly but relatively pain-free.

I'd always been pragmatic enough to realise that because of my awkward gait and dilapidated body, something was going to have to give sometime. When my back injury arrived, it caused another meltdown in my head, to go with the burning sensation in my back every time I tried to walk. However, living on my own, I had the environment to cope, to sulk without anybody having to bear witness to my mood swings. I was solo, stag, solitary, a hermit. I was happy like this in my own little apartment in Kildare Town, with Nigel as my chauffeur whenever we needed each other. Going downstairs to the Gobán Saor if I needed company.

But now things were different. Now there was no Nigel. There was Helena and soon a baby. My thoughts, understandably, often drifted back to what happened to me. I'd get angry just imagining something similar happening to this still-unborn baby of mine.

There's a lot more education out there now around the dangers of concussion and brain injuries in sport – a bang on the ear raises the red flag much quicker than in my day. Asking a suspected concussed player to play on has been equated with asking a drunk driver whether they're okay to drive. That's a perfect description.

Insurance has improved immeasurably too. If what happened to me in 1989 happened today, there's at least a few hundred thousand euros available to help a family rebuild their life. It still leaves a sour taste in my mouth that my parents had the burden of all my medical expenses and care hoisted on their shoulders. There was no support from the FAI or anyone else, despite my injury happening on a football field. Did the FAI have a duty of care towards me? Do they now? All I know is that I've never heard anything from them. I was only fifteen. A fucking schoolboy. I honestly can't fathom what my parents went through, wondering whether I would live, and if I did, what my, and their, quality of life would be like.

What if I had been left a vegetable? Would Mam have travelled to Dublin every day until they turned the machine off? How would this have affected my siblings at home, being raised by their granny? Would I have been shunted into a nursing home in Navan to see out my days, like some victims of brain injuries these days?

What if I had been left intellectually disabled? Would there have been room for me in St Ultan's, the special needs school on Flower Hill? Ironically, I'm living across the road from it now.

With these thoughts racing through my mind, the idea of becoming a dad myself both thrilled and terrified me. What if I was shite at it?

Dads are supposed to be very physical with their children – to lift them, carry them, throw them up in the air and catch them. They're supposed to be able to simply walk with them hand in hand, or place them on their shoulders. I wouldn't be able to do that. I wouldn't be able to teach them how to ride a bike, to chase after them.

I wouldn't be able to do any of this stuff. How would this affect my relationship with my kids?

Eventually I came to realise that I'd just have to do what I always did. I'd have to adapt.

I'd been doing this ever since my injury in 1989. Constantly adapting. Walking. Adapting. Changing my gait. Adapting. Slowing down. Adapting. Refinding my balance. Adapting. Being bullied. Adapting. However, this new change would require a whole new level of adapting.

The last time I'd had so much responsibility was at the summer camp in '96. But back then, I was much younger, much fitter, and had a great team around me to lean on whenever it became too much. Helena would have to be that whole team for me.

If we were a team, Helena was my Messi. She was my Mick Lyons. The tough that got going for me. But there would be times I'd have to fend for myself, and the thought of that terrified me. What if I dropped the baby? What if I slipped when carrying the baby? What if I injured myself while changing the baby on the counter, and the baby fell to the floor?

I always conducted an internal risk assessment for everything I did – step-by-step plans for every movement since my injury. Every move, every single step, needed deep-rooted thought. Every journey had to have an exact plan in place. An exact destination. Every single step needed exact deliberation. Or else.

The result of not focussing absolutely on every step was always the same: collapsing in an unceremonious heap. It happened frequently – whenever my mind drifted momentarily; whenever there was a sudden gust of wind, or an obstacle that burst into sight too late to avoid. A change in surface. A pebble on the ground. A speck of dust landing in my eye. A fleeting thought.

A simple fucking thought could send me crashing onto the ground. If I took my mind off any aspect of the contours of walking, I'd go down. My every thought had to be about walking, cruising, wobbling, one foot in front of the other. Swinging my left arm for balance. All in sync. If one tiny step was left out, that was it. The repercussions were inevitable. Resign myself to a fall.

So the baby would have to row in with the methods and techniques I'd put in place. Surely they would learn to live with my disability?

All of this had to be considered when buying a travel system. Forget what it looked like. Forget what it cost. I'd have to be comfortable with it, and safe with it. I actually liked the first one we looked at. But, like wedding dresses, you can easily fall in love with the first one, and we both felt it was best to shop around a lot, to do loads of research. I'd require something very sturdy, as I'd be leaning on it for support. Three-wheel buggies were a non-starter – I'd need four for balance and stability. I would also need a heavier buggy for this reason. We tried them out in Smyths until the staff were sick of me.

The Graco travel system, the very first one we'd looked at, was the winner. Black and red trim. Heavier than the rest. Sturdy. Manly even. Munster colours and Manchester United colours. Suited us both. I'd be able to walk easier, slightly further, with this.

I could lift the buggy base in and out of the car by carefully planting my feet and leaning my bum against the car boot. Carefully thought out. Step by step. Constantly thinking. Constantly exhausted. Overusing my body and mind.

But even with risk assessments, the best-laid plans often go awry. Helena was having the baby early. I wasn't ready. Would I ever be? But we sped over to Drogheda's midwifery-led unit. I struggled in the door, up the lift and down the lengthy corridor. Sweating profusely when I arrived, I sat down before I collapsed. Now it was Helena's turn to sweat.

The midwife had a pained expression on her face all throughout Helena's labour. I noticed this. Every time I'd sneak a look at her face at the business end, she was squirming in pain. Was she seeing something that I wasn't? Was she thinking something that I couldn't comprehend? Was there something wrong with our baby? I was too scared to ask her. I had been told to stay at the top end and encourage Helena. Nothing else. No Del-boy antics here. Stay in the zone, the 'say-absolutely-fucking-nothing' zone.

I don't know how I'd have coped if there was something wrong or if my baby had a disability. Despite working alongside kids with severe and profound intellectual disabilities, the idea hadn't occurred to me until now. Until the moment I saw the midwife's stressed expression. Thoughts entered. Such thoughts had already rumbled through Helena's head. She'd seen the kids I work with in the school. Do mothers overthink more than fathers? Probably. A disabled Dad with a disabled child. Surely they'd take the child off me. How could I look after a newborn baby?

But when I was presented with the scissors to cut the umbilical cord I flourished. I could do this no problem, squelchy and all as it was. The wee girl was taken from her mammy and rushed off away from us. Was my overthinking about to be proved correct? Were my fears to be realised?

But then I was handed this tiny, swaddled, cleaned up bundle. I had to sit down to hold her for the first time. Being up most of the night meant my legs were more like jelly than ever before. The pain in my hips was burning. My back was on fire.

But my baby. My Eileen. She was perfect.

I gazed into her eyes and I forgot about my disability for a few minutes. I was not in pain, for the first time in twenty years.

The midwife was free now for questioning. I asked her about her pained expression throughout Helena's labour. A toothache. Well fuck me. Could she not have told me at the start?

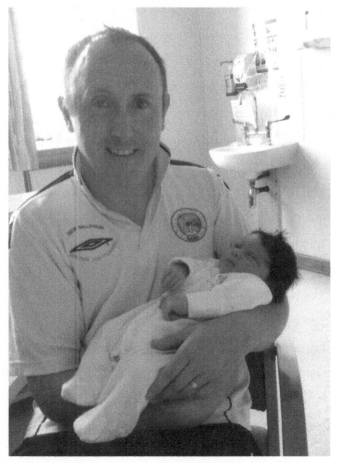

I'm a father!

My attention turned back to Eileen. Here was the most important thing in my life now. She took my breath away. I was stunned. I was a dad. I wasn't disabled. I was without thought for a few moments. Just looking into her eyes. I could have ran a marathon at that moment. The adrenaline rush. The hopes. The dreams. The absolute fear.

I drove home on my own that evening. In a daze. In a dream. I stopped into a local pub for a bite to eat. The Round O, where this journey all began. I'd come full circle. I just stared at my dinner and picked at it. Friends came over to congratulate me. I was away with the fairies, baffled.

Bringing Eileen home was an incredible experience. We stopped at Zucchinis for dinner. We were bringing home a new human being. Somebody we'd have to care for, love and cherish. Despite being disabled, I knew I could manage this. Of course I could do this. I had no choice. Gooch adored her.

More adaptation was required. Moses baskets, one upstairs and one downstairs. Helena could carry the child with absolute safety up or down the stairs. Hence the need for a Moses basket both upstairs and downstairs.

The safest and most pain-free way for me to get the baby to bed was to carry the Moses basket in my left hand up the stairs, leaning on my right hand on the bannister. With the weight on my left leg, I could gently push off every step with the baby cradled in the basket. Whenever I stumbled, instinct gave me a split second to place the Moses basket gently on a step and fall directly behind the baby to prevent the fall downstairs. Because my grip was still firmly on the bannister I regained composure fairly quickly and carried on.

Once upstairs, my hand would then balance my weight against the wall until I got to the bedroom door. Placing the Moses basket into the cot,

I could then lean my stomach against the bed rail and transfer the baby from the basket into the cot.

Then I'd tip-toe out and clamber back down the stairs as quietly as my noisy and awkward gait allowed. I'd be petrified that I'd wake Eileen and have to clamber back up the stairs all over again.

Getting the baby down the stairs involved a different technique. I'd come down on my bum, cradling the baby in my lap, covered with my right hand for safety, the other hand clutching the bannister. Bumming down step by precarious step.

Transferring the precious treasure under my left arm once again, as careful as Peter Stringer protecting the rugby ball. Next, composing myself, the thought of standing up. My spindly, giraffe-like legs steadying themselves, my very weak glutes firing into action, clambering up to grab onto the wall, with my right hand spread as wide as possible to balance the extra load.

Everything had to be perfect to make it work. The consequences of a fall with the baby in my arms didn't bear thinking about. I had to be extremely careful, every time.

As Eileen grew up, in the blink of an eye, Helena and I spoke about having a second. We didn't have to think about it too long, and pretty soon she was pregnant again. This time, it was a boy.

I'd always wondered what having a boy would be like. Would he be very different from me? I was an adventurer as a toddler and as a young boy. Always roaming around and curious. Always searching for adventure. Would I now get to see how I'd have turned out if I hadn't been injured?

As the children have grown older, I've grown with them. They've adapted to me and my ways of doing things, my ways of going places, my ways of living. Helena helped Eileen learn to ride a bike and, at three years of age,

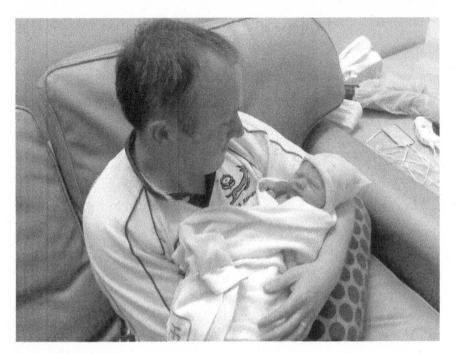

I'm a father again!

Joey was climbing on a bike way beyond his years. He *is* a mini-me in many ways. A great climber, very inquisitive, always testing. He loves dogs and sport, and adores exploring and adventures.

He was in his stroller until he was four. Not because he needed it, but because I did, even for a walk of the shortest distance. I needed his weight in it to walk further. The stroller was absolutely no good without him in it, too light and unstable. Of course, soon I was overthinking again. Would this affect Joe in the long term? Would it affect him, having been in a stroller way longer than he needed to be?

'Daddy, when your leg is better next year, I won't need the buggy.'

'Daddy, won't you be able to ride a bike with me next year when your leg gets better?'

'Daddy, can we go on a long walk next year when your leg gets better?'

How can I say no? And yet, I can't possibly say yes. How do I tell the kids about my brain injury? They think I got injured playing football and just hurt my leg and my toe. I'm a firm believer in age-appropriate information. Ideally, I'd like to paint the picture that, although I've been through an awful lot, I'm fine, I adore being their Daddy and I hope they'll tell me if they're being made to feel bad because of my disability. I still hope I'll embarrass them, because that's a real father's job!

How will they cope with finding out that their dad had a severe brain injury? I'll have to ensure I give them the tools to cope, to be able to brush it off with humour. They slag me off these days, which I always find amusing and I encourage it.

'Mammy, we'd be able to go on 'Ireland's Fittest Family', but Daddy would have to stay at home!' Joe said.

I laughed and then Helena replied, 'Of course Daddy would come; he'd be our biggest and loudest cheerleader!'

JUNE 2016 – TWENTY-SEVEN YEARS AFTER THE INJURY

A letter to my brother:

Dear James,

There are only a few select people I've ever 'let in', because I don't want to alienate myself by being a moan. These people can empathise with what I'm going through, but really have no idea what pain I'm in and the gravity of the issues I'm fighting daily. You are one of these people, since you've left for Hong Kong.

This bloody midlife crisis has been going on for a couple of years on and off. Questioning everything, being pissed off with every little thing (even more so than usual!). It doesn't help that I'm sitting here with a broken hip from falling on the beach.

How a football concussion left me disabled for life. How my two-year-old son is far better at walking than I am. He's more stable, much faster, and lives without fear of falling. I spend every moment just concentrating on staying straight, keeping myself safe, and trying not to fall.

I often wonder, if Navan hospital had been better equipped with a CT scanner, might I have been rushed straight to Beaumont instead of the delay in Our Lady's, waiting for an ambulance? Was this the only reason I was kept in casualty for so long – waiting for an ambulance to become available? Were the experts in the hospital aware of the gravity of my situation? With the concussion, was 'talk and die syndrome' occurring? If I was still unconscious, as I was in the team bus, would the people responsible have hurried up an ambulance? Surely precious time was being lost while the blood clot grew and spread and did increasing damage?

But I know Navan Hospital saved my life too. If they had not sent me to Beaumont, if they'd sent me home with a few disprin, I'd have died. So I'm thankful to them too.

I'm very anxious about the future. I realise I can do absolutely nothing about the future but try to plan it and work around what happens when a situation arises. But I've always been a logical thinker, a deep thinker, an overthinker (which doesn't bloody help).

The fulcrum of it all is the state of my body, I think. Basically once I start feeling pain again, the fear of it is worse than the actual pain. I can deal with a lot of pain – micro pain, macro pain, chronic pain. I've been off Difene for probably two years now and have been managing the pain ever since with an improved physio regime, but had to take one last week when my knee went. It fixed itself over about thirty-six hours and the sky was a little brighter then. But the fear surrounds me, the fear consumes me, envelops me, scares the fuck out of me.

I won't lie though. The 'fear' is something much more serious than even that. It consumes me wholeheartedly; the darkest of clouds over my head the whole time. This fear goes straight to my head and I suddenly start thinking: What if the pain gets worse? What if I can't work anymore? What if I can't provide for my family anymore? What if I can't contribute to society? The panic that sets in when I feel a twinge or a dart of pain is all-consuming. It sends me into overdrive.

It kills me, and yet I don't really say anything – except this letter, of course. I feel it's best to just 'sulk' and tell nobody, because I don't want to drag any-body into the hole I've dug for myself.

I've always tried to put on a public smiling face – 'Sure I'm grand.' Nobody probes, nobody questions, nobody wants to bloody hear me com-plaining. I don't want to complain. I've learned to fight this alone, I've had to learn to be strong. I'm used to running on empty and have taught myself through experience that working it all out by myself is the best way for me.

At work, I'm the happy-go-lucky wobbler who just gets on with the job, loves the kids I'm working with and gets on well with the staff.

There was one night that really stands out to me. I was driving down to Thomond in January, a trip that did loads to lift my spirits. I had 'Stand Up and Fight' on repeat all the way down and I screamed my lungs out. But the fire in my knees and hips could have melted the Lambert Glacier.

The trip meant so much to me. I was going stag, dodging snow. I made Limerick in loads of time and walked across the back of the terrace to the TV broadcasters' area. I was met with a firm handshake by Alan Quinlan [no relation], and he introduced me to the rest of the TV team. He told them about my injury and they were probing, genuinely interested in hearing about me. I stumbled back towards the terrace where I'd stand for the rest of the day and managed to watch the whole squad warming up against Stade Français. Leaning against the barrier, I was screaming and shouting, venting and channelling my anger properly. My knee went on me in the second half, exhausted from the walk and standing against the barrier. Luckily, I had spoken to the medic at the corner of the pitch on his medical buggy before kickoff.

He understood and told me to climb aboard. He dropped me back to my car in LIT car park next door. The slagging I got from all the walkers following us was unreal. I still smile at that. More black humour. Then, more than ever, rugby and Munster felt like an umbilical cord that would always tie me back to Limerick.

Months later, after I'd broken my hip, Axel Foley told me via Facebook messenger to get myself a decent physio programme and I'd be in line for selection in September. Whether he was bigging me up or slagging me off, it didn't matter. It was an incredible boost for me that he'd actually take time out to reply to me.

Some people, very close to me since my injury, only see my leg as the issue. This disappoints me, but that's life. They think it's as simple as that. It's like they have a PhD in disability studies. They don't see any other issues, for them that's all that's wrong with me. It's probably my fault, because I don't groan, complain or bother correcting them. Perhaps they aren't overly concerned with me; they have their own issues. I'm my own man now and have my own life. Am I better off being my own therapist?

What they don't see is that something as simple as the wind can be my worst enemy. It last happened outside the credit union, when I exited the car, lost my stability and collapsed on the ground, injuring my wrist badly. An onlooker asked if I needed any help, but I said I was perfecting a stunt for an upcoming movie. He was happy with that.

The fatigue I feel every day is extreme, and people don't see this either. Even Hel gets pissed off with me when I fall asleep at 7pm most nights after my physio, because she's wide awake, just finished work. I'm using seventy-five percent more energy than a fully able-bodied person to do absolutely simple things, and it's taking a huge toll on my ravaged body. I'm awake at 6am most mornings because I've always gone to bed early, but the efforts I've made during the day really take a lot out of me.

If you can imagine the worst hangover you've ever had and the tiredness that came with it – minus the nausea – that comes close to how I feel every day. Part of it comes from the constant thinking and analysing. Always trying to work out the safest way to get around. Always trying to pre-empt the journey, no matter how short, to make sure I don't fall to pieces. What can I grab onto along the way to avoid collapsing? It's never as simple as going from A to B. There are so many variables involved, it's more like going from A to Z just to get to B.

Perhaps on some level I have also gone through a grieving process for the body I once had, that was so cruelly taken away from me. It has been hard coming to terms with what I was left with, after being so fit. However, whenever I have met parents of people who died young, I have felt a certain amount of guilt. Did they think, 'Why wasn't my son, at least, left like Phil?'

I hope I haven't too harsh on Helena above. She remains the best person I've ever met. But marriage can be downright frustrating at times, especially when kids come along. Her job is one of the most frustrating things for me. She's supposed to finish at 5pm every day, but it's often much later.

She would often not be home until after eight. The feeling of dread when I get the frequent text that simply says 'late'. I need her to be home so much to take the kids up to bed.

I know she can't control it, but the fact is that I can't switch off until she's home or the kids are comfortably in bed. I'm just about coping with the kids, but the 'late' text seems to be coming more frequently.

Speaking of the kids, I keep thinking about what happens if my disability starts to affect them. I'm looking forward to the day when I can bring them to school, but can't stop worrying: What if I fall on the way and all their classmates start laughing and slagging them off? It's one thing if I'm being slagged off about my wobble, but I don't want my kids taking the hit. I'd like to educate them to be just as blasé about my disability as I am. So if they get slagged at school, they can laugh it off just as I do now.

They are the reason I get myself out of bed every day, despite the agony. I feel I must show them that I have a wee bit of pride and self-respect, and I can get up to work every day. I need to feel I'm contributing.

The kids are brilliant, but they are also the biggest challenge at this stage of my life. To see them smiling at me when I get down to play with them, to see their faces when I'm reading them a story (and they do love stories), to see them simply growing up, going through their different life stages.

But they really wear me out. If I'm preparing dinner, I have to give them a bollocking if they even look like they might come near the kitchen. I guard it with my life for their lives. Carrying a boiling-hot pan from the hob over to the sink to empty the boiling water is an immense challenge, though it's a distance of only three feet. Even the dog knows how difficult this is for me and stays away. I've fallen a couple of times in a heap, with boiling spuds all over the floor.

I don't get out much, but, to be honest, I'm absolutely wiped out come 7pm every evening, only fit to do my physio and zonk out on the sofa. Getting out and doing something outside of the family may help the way I'm feeling, but I'm not sure exactly what to do. Is my life coping with the kids good for me or should I make the effort to get out for a pint of a weekend? Or something else? Dad had training twice a week and match days when he was my age. Obviously I can't do anything like that.

And that's life at the moment in a nutshell, Bro. Keep it to yourself please. Looking forward to going for a pint with you over Easter and chatting a bit more.

For now, I'm off to bed,

Love you,

Phil

APRIL 2021 – THIRTY-ONE YEARS AFTER THE INJURY

Eileen has come in from the back garden. She's hurt herself. Again.

She's eight now, young enough that in any other child, the first reaction might be to curl up their lip and cry. But Eileen's brain processes pain differently to your average kid, as she suffers from childhood fainting. This is not related to my brain injury at all; a paediatrician has told us that it's quite common and hopefully she'll grow out of it. But it's still scary as a parent.

You see, when Eileen experiences pain, she faints and starts shivering, almost like a seizure. About ten seconds later, she comes through, groggy but fine.

Today she has arrived into the kitchen from the back garden, the scab on her elbow from a previous fall after bursting from a hurley. It's sending a trickle of blood down her arm, but on the whole she seems okay. As I wash the blood off, she says she's not in any pain. I turn to the counter to grab another plaster, because she's fidgeting with the one I've already pulled out. As I turn around, her eyes close, her head tilts back and she falls backwards, her head hitting the tiles. Crack.

As quickly as my broken body allows me, I'm kneeling beside her, cradling her. I curse myself. I reacted so slowly, it was like I was moving through jam. I couldn't react. Any other father would have caught her and lowered her safely to the ground, I tell myself. She was just a couple of feet from me as she fell.

But no, I just stood there, watching it happen in slow motion. Crack.

Kneeling beside her, I'm petrified. That was such a belt on the back of the head. My mind races. Fleeting memories swirl of everything that happened to me. Visions of Eileen in an ambulance. Eileen in a coma. Eileen with a brain injury.

I hold her head. I tell her over and over again how sorry I am. How useless I am as a father. How could I let that happen? How could I let my child collapse and bang her head like that? How could I ever forgive myself for that sound? Crack.

Helena comes running down stairs. Just seconds have passed, but it feels like hours. I burst out crying. I tell her what happened, how useless I am. But what could I do? None of the usual signs were there. She reacted really well to the cut. No tears, no complaining. None of the usual signs. But then: Crack.

She moved so slowly as she fell; like the canopy of a giant redwood finally seeing its roots again, centuries after last meeting. I should have known she'd faint. A real father would have.

Helena tries to calm me down, but I'm a mess of snot and tears. You're a fucking eejit. You're a fucking eejit. You're a fucking eejit. I repeat it over and over again in my head. Eventually Eileen comes round and I gather myself together. Ultimately, she's fine. And I finally come to learn that I'm fine too, even if that sickening sound haunts me to this day. Crack.

I can't react like other dads. This body isn't built for speed anymore. But both my kids are happy. Both my kids are healthy and loved, with a safe space to call home. And they love their dad as much as he loves them.

I can't really ask for any more than that, can I?

CHAPTER 16

THE WALK OF LIFE

8 DECEMBER 1989 – TWO WEEKS AFTER THE INJURY

There was always a lot of slagging between the Torro lads and Parkvilla. It would be Torro's cup final game, 'cause that Parkvilla side was so far ahead of everyone else in Navan.

I cycled to the game. It was very foggy, and maybe because of that we had very few players on our sideline. Just enough lads to play the match really.

I don't know whether I actually remember what happened, or if, over the years, I've made myself remember it.

To be honest, it didn't seem that bad at the time. Phil came into the dugout on our side – there was a home and away dugout on the same side. I knew, after the referee stopped the game, there was something up. But I wasn't too worried until half time, when I saw the panic in Phil's dugout.

We didn't have mobile phones in those days. So I didn't find out what happened immediately afterwards. I cycled home. Gordon, one of my teammates, rang me that evening to say Phil was in hospital. But it wasn't really until school the next day when we found out what was happening. Father Gabriel was brilliant, he was the line of contact between us and Phil.

I went up to Phil's house not long after the injury. I went up in a little blue car from school. And I was a ball of sweat. I was that nervous. There were a lot of people around the house and I just wanted to get in and get out.

A few of the townie lads gave me awful grief for what happened. 'Here comes the murderer,' they'd say. They were only slagging, I think. They knew it was an accident. But I do remember them saying it.

Ray Kealy, Torro United player

P iecing together what happened on that fateful day in 1989, and the threads that spin out from a foggy football pitch in Navan to Sydney, New York and beyond has left me with a lot of time for reflection. And one conclusion I've come to is that Ireland, in my opinion, is one of the worst places in the world, attitude-wise, in which to be disabled.

I've seen how flippant and blasé people in other countries are regarding the disabled, and maybe it's their directness that I'm comfortable with. They stare quickly, but ask questions in a very mannerly way. Once I tell them it's a football injury, they shrug their shoulders and that's it – problem solved, issue sorted, awkwardness avoided, move on. 'Ahhh, you're Irish; tell me something Irish!' This has always been my experience on my travels.

In Irish towns and villages, disgust or pity is what I've encountered. Even in big cities I'm not safe. The taxi man who brought me across the Liffey only wanted his bigger pound of flesh back in the day. Empathy my arse. People here pussy foot around me.

Sure, I might get an awkward smile if I catch them chancing a swift stare. But even when they avert their gaze rapidly, I see it and laugh inside. Are they uncomfortable because they can see the pain I'm in trying to walk? Are they mortified because of how I look? Are they afraid and concerned because they can see my speed wobbles and the threat of me about to collapse?

I've always found that children see me, while adults just notice me.

The Irish are very British in their outlook on disabilities. I know they'll probably not want to hear this, but in my experience it's true. Telling their kids not to stare; instilling the hangups their own parents handed down to them. For me, this is the worst way to encourage children to embrace the differences that disabled people bring. Surely a simple wave, salute or 'How's she cuttin'?' would show children that it's no big deal if someone is using a crutch to wobble along or is in a wheelchair.

More often than not, my wobbling or shuffling means I'm equated with a drunk guy or a bloke off his head on drugs. I can sit on one drink for the whole night and still walk out of the pub looking like I've had a wild time.

I noticed something the first time I used a power chair in the Trafford shopping centre in Manchester. I struggled with the long distance of the centre – the mobility shop was further away than I'd hoped. When I was wobbling along, I pointed out that it seemed stupid to stick the mobility shop at a hard-to-reach entrance, rather than in the middle of the centre where it's easier to access. Of course, all I received was the same, sorry-for-your-loss-stares that I've been getting for decades.

But when I used a power chair, it was like I'd snuck into a telephone box, stripped off and started wearing my underpants over my tights. People were so much more accepting once they saw me using a recognised device. It was like I was a new man, superhero status bestowed on me by my extra fast supercar.

A power chair. Such a simple thing, which turned judging looks into empathetic smiles, salutes, sneaky shake-the-head-winks. People were all over me immediately, opening doors and helping me reach the top shelf of the shop. I was special, I was Superman. A Superman who needed help, but Superman nonetheless. It seemed that they didn't need to know *why* I needed the device. They just recognised the device.

Part of me wonders if the power chair made it clearer that I didn't have an intellectual disability. Surely I couldn't, if I was able to navigate, at speed, this motorised vehicle? Did this make people understand, at last, that only my legs were damaged? Was this the object that they required to understand my needs?

The question then arises, why do able-bodied people need this security blanket? It's the disabled person they should be looking out for, not the device that helps with the disability.

It's exactly the same in Ireland.

Too many 'normal' people automatically think that just because a person has a physical disability, then they must also have an intellectual disability. They don't necessarily go hand-in-hand. In fact, they often don't. Educate yourselves. There's a mountain of information out there. Google it.

What is it that disgusts them? Is it that I'm sweating profusely, constantly wheezing as I try to catch my breath, saving speed wobbles along the way, readying myself to land in a crumpled heap on the ground? Ironically, if I try to stretch out my gait, to walk more 'normally' – even for a tiny bit – my leg becomes cocky, laughs at me, and I collapse in a heap.

It's not just other people's thoughts. It's actions too. Every day, I have to live with disabled parking bays being abused, because they're easy to park in. There's a fucking reason they're easy and *accessible* to park in. Excuses I've heard over the years include:

'Sure, I'll only be a minute!'

'It's late at night now, so no disabled driver would be out!'

'Nobody will know!'

'It's raining and I don't want to get wet!'

'Sure, there are plenty more for the poor disabled drivers close by!'

Some don't even bother to make an excuse; they just park in these places because it suits them. Are they just lazy fuckers, or do they see disabled drivers as lazy fuckers?

Taxis are among the worst offenders. Many of them just don't give a shite. There is a disabled parking bay attached to a taxi rank on the square in Navan, and I've lost track of the number of times I've had to beep them politely out of it. Most of them move on. Most.

I had an interesting debate with one taxi man who was parked in the disabled parking bay and just wouldn't move. He told me it was a designated parking bay for the bus stop across the road. 'So why are you parked in it?' I countered. He suddenly changed his tune, and then came up with what he thought would be a winner: 'It's the disabled parking bay for the boy who lives above the shop.' Who knew Meath County Council could afford to give disabled people bespoke parking spots?

My folks arrived and tried to engage him, but he wasn't for moving. This was years ago, but the parking bay he was sure he was okay to idle in is still being abused daily.

Of course, it's not only taxi drivers. I've been to events all around the country, to stadiums being used for festivals, football tournaments and the like. And the registration tents are nearly always set up in the best and handiest place – the disabled parking bays. You couldn't make it up. And really, why would you want to?

Of course, they're more polite about it than some.

'We'll find you another parking spot, you'll be grand.' Surely you'll be happy with the crumbs from the table? Disabled people, always the afterthought. We'll see what we've left and then we'll see if we can afford to make it accessible to the disabled.

I'm not sure if Brown Thomas still has those orange discs placed strategically on the disabled parking bay. The first time I used their car park, I hadn't a clue what it was. Once I got out of the car, the orange disc sprang into action and a loud, recorded message told the whole car park that this parking bay was *only* to be used for accredited disabled drivers. Genius, I thought.

The abuse of these designated parking spots is one example of the absolute disregard, lack of education and sheer ignorance that exists in Irish society. I'm honestly not sure the fines or penalties are tough enough. It might be the only way people will learn – if they're hit in the pocket.

I had a blazing argument in the Keadeen Hotel sauna years ago. One of the punters, who didn't know me, came in and started telling a story about how he had recently injured his ankle and secured himself a disabled parking badge for two years. I hopped off him, telling him how ignorant this was – did he not feel guilty, pretending to have a disability?

'Sure, I'm not the only one doing it,' came his meek reply.

I met him recently, when I returned to the Keadeen after fifteen years' absence. I slagged him off about his indiscretion years previously. He was mortified, because the sauna was full this time.

I've tried to use humour when I encounter parking bay violations. I've even screamed out my window: 'Congratulations. I'm delighted it worked!'

They turn around and ask, smiling, 'What worked?'

I pause for a millisecond and then say, 'Lourdes!'

And while I usually receive a big 'fuck off', it's they who slink away, mortified, to laughter from bystanders.

Sometimes people fight back too. One brave soul summoned up the cojones one evening in Clane, as I stood leaning against the car, stretching after a long drive.

'There's nothing wrong with you,' he said.

As quick as I could, and with a huge grin, I answered, 'Listen, mate, I know it's kind of unbelievable that a bloke this good-looking could actually be disabled, but it's true!'

He wasn't expecting that. He swore like a sailor and walked back to his car. He stayed in his driver's seat for a good two minutes watching me. As soon as my legs were ready, my brain told them to move, and off I shuffled. I could still feel him staring at me, and then I heard it:

'If you're disabled, where's your fucking wheelchair?'

He's not alone. Evidently, I don't look disabled enough for certain randomers. Because I'm not crippled to the nth degree, and I can wobble about, apparently for some this means I shouldn't be eligible for a blue parking card.

Why does using a wheelchair, or another mobility aid, put people so much more at ease than watching me struggle to keep my balance with my awkward gait and ugly stance? I want to maintain a small semblance of fitness, rather than becoming increasingly reliant on a power chair. Is that my problem or theirs? If I resigned myself to using the chair full-time, I would probably also have to find a new job, a desk job, just to appease these people.

Of course, I have positive experiences sometimes. Once, in Clontarf Castle, as I approached the counter, the head porter or junior manager engaged me a few steps ahead. I enquired if there was somewhere I could watch the match and perhaps get some grub. He ushered me towards the Knights Bar and, as I turned, not exactly on a sixpence, he wondered out loud: 'Do you need any wheels, sir?'

I was stunned. I'd never been asked this question before. A huge grin appeared on my face and I replied, 'No thank you, but thanks a million for the offer. I really appreciate it, but I need to get the steps in.'

He shot back with a 'very good, sir,' and off I meandered.

What made him different? Was he more educated in life? Did he have an elderly relative who struggled with their mobility? Was I the first disabled punter he'd ever come across? Did he have to dig deep and face his fears, throwing the gauntlet down and waiting for me to pick it up? It could have been an awkward moment for both of us. But he asked and gave me the agency to decline. And I was delighted with that.

Other places are making an effort too. Zucchini's restaurant in Navan have installed a chair lift up to their restaurant. It's not just for me, but it's a marvellous idea, which invites elderly or less mobile people to travel in comfort, especially after a steak meal.

I feel sorriest for the parents of kids born with a disability. Firstly, they have to suffer the stigma of having a baby with a disability. Despite what you'd hope, this is still very real in Ireland. It's changing. Slowly. Very slowly.

Secondly, they have to battle for services and equipment, assessments and everything else that can make their lives and their children's lives less stressful. The movement of SLTs, physios and OTs from town to town, never lasting long anywhere, means that this crucial time in a child's life, when they could be learning lots, can be a succession of missed opportunities.

Because of some pen pusher or bean counter's need to continually swap staff around, kids lose out and parents pull their hair out.

If you're reading this and thinking I'm wrong, look around you. Just look at the recent cases where not every child in the country was afforded a school place, because of disabilities. Parents have essentially been told by the State that their kids would be better off at home. Out of sight. Hidden away from society.

Every child deserves an education. And every child that can be, should be integrated into 'normal' schools. It's crucial for mainstream children to interact and ask their childhood questions, to see that it's okay to be different, that it's okay to ask for help and that it's okay to offer help.

In most of the countries I've travelled to, the first thing people ask is, 'What happened to your leg?'

And then I answer them, and that's it. We both move on. I can't wait for the day when that happens in Ireland too.

I believe that integration from a young age is hugely important in educating kids. It's like early intervention – the earlier you realise your child has a problem, the exponentially better. Early education, like intervention, makes lots of sense to me. Give kids dolls in wheelchairs; let Action Man walk with a crutch – he has been through a few wars after all. Barbie and Ken might motor on with a power chair, as they're getting on a bit at this stage.

Kids will learn quicker if they're exposed to these things at a young age. It will become the norm. Kids' TV shows now have characters in wheelchairs. 'Fireman Sam' has a character who cruises around in her wheelchair doing keepie-uppies with footballs – she's a normal eleven-year-old kid who everyone accepts.

Maybe children need to educate their parents on how easy it is to become comfortable with the subject of disabilities? We've tried educating the parents for generations, with little success. Let's change tack – let's bypass the older, prehistoric generations, and focus on the more important children of today.

Eileen is a fantastic football player, the top scorer in her team. In her first match as U12 captain, she notched a hat-trick in a 3-2 win. But at another game, I spotted a young boy on the sidelines, 'stimming', with headphones on. Obviously not too interested in sitting and watching the match, he was allowed to roam about. Joe spied the young chap and asked if he had autism. I answered possibly, and ushered him over to chat. He was a bit hesitant at first. I told Joe to pretend to try to lift a big tractor tyre nearby, and to ask without talking, just using gestures, for some help. The bigger boy accepted Joe's invite when Joe put on a stressed face while trying to lift the tyre. However, once he realised the weight of it, he baulked, dropped the tyre immediately and walked off, saying, 'Too heavy.'

Joe persisted and sidled over to him, introducing himself. He got a name back, and they chatted about favourite colours, movies and food until the match finished and we left. Hopefully we'll meet Tom again at another match. Joe is now forearmed with how he'll be with his next meet.

I used my power chair recently on a visit to Joe's class. The kids all stared, and one shouted out, 'He brought his Batmobile!'

Everyone burst out laughing, though slightly nervously, unsure of what the teacher thought. Simply put, it was brilliant. Suddenly the kids were all at ease. A genius ice-breaker. That's all that's needed. Humour. Because of that experience, twenty-six children probably won't have a hang up when they next see someone using an aid.

Ultimately, unless you're immediately affected by disability, you don't have to give a damn. Why the long delay in fully ratifying the UN Convention on the Rights of Persons with Disabilities? Opened for signature in 2007, but only ratified by Ireland in 2018. Was it too much hassle?

It shouldn't take someone close to you being disabled for you to give a shit about disabilities. Maybe there are a few politicians who are genuine, but overall, our priorities leave a lot to be desired.

The old adage of 'he who shouts loudest gets heard' has a lot of truth to it. However, it's an absolute crime that a parent needs to fight so hard and so loudly for what should be basic human rights. Surely society should look after its most vulnerable with more empathy?

AN END HAS A START

JUNE 2022 – THIRTY-TWO YEARS AFTER THE INJURY

'So, Daddy, did it work?'

Those are the words of my son Joe when I get home from DCU after trying out their new robotic exoskeleton. He was hoping I'd be fixed. I can see the heartbreak on his face when he realises I'm still walking with a limp. He's stuck with me holding on to his neck for balance when we walk anywhere.

This happens a lot, both Joe and Eileen wondering when their Daddy will be fixed. I wonder about it myself. I've wondered about it since I was confined to my bedroom in Navan after the injury, with nothing but a computer as my best friend.

I taught myself how to write a few simple programmes using BASIC. I learned how to touch-type. I sat there, writing, constantly hoping, constantly wondering, constantly anxious about what the future held. However, what always comforted me were the dreams I had. Dreams of travelling. Dreams of getting better. Dreams of running.

In that bedroom, I learned to love reading. To love the places it could take you and the people you could meet. I wonder now about my own story, and how it might possibly end.

Will it be a story I can share with my kids, so they'll grow up with empathy? Will they realise that I'd go without everything to give them anything. Though they've missed out on some of the things that other fathers can do, like throwing them up into the air or carrying them on their shoulders, I hope they know that this cranky old man loves them dearly and will do anything he can to ensure they have a good upbringing and a happy life. I get a huge lift when Joe, beeping like a reversing truck, arrives alongside me when he sees I need his shoulder, and lets me lean on his neck to walk along.

'Daddy, do you ever worry that what happened to you will happen to me?' he asks as we're strolling through Blanchardstown Shopping Centre. Me in my power chair and his hand on top of mine. I adore it when they hold my hand.

In my head I'm worried sick, but I can't tell him that.

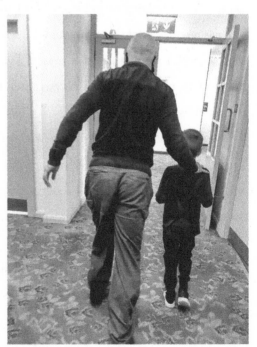

Joe lends a helping shoulder.

'Son, you're a *far* better player than I was ever going to be; you're too clever a footballer …'

Ironically, Joey's U-7 Parkvilla team have met Torro Utd a couple of times. One time they beat them 7-0, with Joey scoring a hat-trick; another, they beat them in the final of the Kells Tournament, and my seven-year-old notched a brace.

Hopefully they'll love their dad as much as my dad's kids love him. I am immensely proud of them both.

Is this a story for my parents, who've been so intrinsic in rehabbing me for years? They were there when I needed a hand on the shoulder and when I needed a kick in the arse. They helped me get back to school, find a job, a house, become the man they always wanted me to be. Even if I had to move at a slightly slower pace than any of us could have imagined.

Would it be a story for Helena, who sees beyond the limp, the brain injury, the pains and the fatigue and who loves me because of who I am, not in spite of it? I hope she realises how big a difference she makes to my life every single day. Like the time I won a Simon Zebo competition for two tickets to Ireland versus Australia. Helena screamed in delight, but I was immediately terrified: How was I going to get to my seat? How would I get from the DART station? How would we get back to the car from the stadium? I brought a crutch with me and thankfully, as soon as the stewards saw a recognised device, they ushered me through a shortcut, rather than the meandering queue back to the platform. But that's the nature of Helena – always looking for the silver lining while I'm checking to see if there are any disabled parking spots nearby. Thanks Zeebs.

Would it be a story for the powers that be in the FAI? Why didn't they reach out to my parents at the time, or at any time since? It's not as if I was in a car crash, or had been diagnosed with cancer as a young foot-baller. I got injured playing the game they promote, left disabled from the game they spend a fortune on advertising. I was one of their own. Would they set a precedent by reaching out to me? Surely it would have been the empathetic thing to do, as the parent company, even in those days. Are they simply an old boys' club that has no thought of player welfare?

Aside from Gerry Browne and Peter McManus, who were heavily involved with the club and were in regular contact, I was never approached by anyone in the FAI. My parents did receive a heart-warming letter from Des Clancy, father of the current (2022) St Patrick's Athletic manager, along with other communications from friends and relatives which I still have in my scrapbook.

Same with the referees' association. Nothing.

FIFA really needs to get a grip on themselves regarding concussion. I'm still not convinced they give a shit. Players are constantly being let play on during international tournaments despite enduring nasty brain injuries.

Would this be a story to help Irish people cope with disability better? To help improve attitudes to disability? When people see me these days in a shopping centre, using a shopping trolley as a zimmer frame or a power chair to negotiate my way around, they are much more comfortable with that than if they see me moving around without an aid. But what they don't realise is that, once the trolley is gone, I'm back struggling like a toddler in a wind tunnel until I get to the car. Where, hopefully, I can hit reset.

People simplistically think it's just my leg that's the issue, that if my leg was fixed my problems would be over. Unfortunately, my brain injury is more complex than that. Balance is another huge challenge, and confidence in my ability to stay upright for any length of time. The mood swings have dissipated a lot, largely due to some of the pains fading. My kids have become a lot more independent, which also helps me immeasurably. They have started to realise that they can help me hugely by inviting me to grab onto their shoulders, just like Helena does.

My self-deprecating sense of humour has broken down a few barriers with people who are freaked out by my disability. People tend to think that because I walk like a drunk and talk like a drunk, I must be a drunk! I like changing people's minds.

Would this be a story for other disabled people? To show them that the sky's the limit. Sheer determination and a hard neck have got me where I am today despite the hand I was dealt. I'm not sure the pre-injury me would have answered an advert in the *Sydney Morning Herald*: 'Australian actor seeks Irish person to practice accent with. Will pay. Galway preferred.'

Ryan Johnson was going to play a part in *The Beauty Queen of Leenane*. He paid $20 an hour to listen to my rambling stories so that he could record and perfect the accent. I brought a Galway girl to the opening night and, as soon as she heard him, she whispered a bit too loudly, 'We don't speak like that in Galway!'

'Ssshhh, don't tell him!'

I had had to teach myself how to talk again years previously, and I laughed a little inside at this.

I had a chip on my shoulder for years, and I became paranoid whenever anybody crossed the street as I wobbled towards them. I wasn't the easiest to get on with. I was cantankerous and bitter. I thought everything was everybody else's fault, as it couldn't be me. Years later though, I now realise it was me. It was all me. The chronic pain made me this way.

Would this be a story for the great men I've learned to surround myself with? Dad, James, Ken, Padraig, Hank, Denis, Paul, Mickey, Luke and others. These are go-to guys, stand-up guys. Always with a grin on their faces. Always making me laugh. We share the same brand of black humour.

Hank Traynor was a great friend in college and a huge crutch for me. On one occasion, we left our accommodation together on a very icy and steep driveway. There was no way I could have made it safely down the slope and onto the path. Hank linked me and basically held me upright as he commentated on us going down the slope. I had to contend with the slope, the ice and fits of laughter that I couldn't stop. 'We'll make the Winter Olympics yet, Philly!'

Hank was part of the Meath side that won the All Ireland football title in 1999, and he sorted me tickets for each of the games, including the final. He'd always cajole me and 'big me up' in front of friends, and his gregariousness was always uplifting.

Would it be a story for the women in my life? Mam. How can I ever thank her for all she did? Mam gave up her life for three and a half months to sit by my bedside and make me her 100% focus. Then she had to go home and give more to my siblings. She was a constant I needed at the time. When I escaped from hospital, she then had to rear me again, as a teenager with toddler feet and a toddler's emotional intelligence.

But not just her. Both my grannies stepped right up. As did big Barbara next door, Valerie, Bridie, Margaret, Marian and all my aunts, especially Liz.

And Helena ... Always Helena.

Would it be a story for my Parkvilla team-mates, to show them how close I came to dying? Their antics that day never sat well with me, but talking to some of them since I can see they didn't understand how serious it all was.

Would this be a story for those who looked after me over the years? I've met up with some of the staff from Beaumont Hospital who cared for me so unselfishly during early 1990. Bernie and Liz, I'll be forever in your debt. Carole, you've done more than you could ever imagine.

Brian Kennedy was very good to me. I was probably the first disabled student he had ever encountered. When I trained under Marian in the school office, he indulged me and my idea to raise money for the school sports fund with my Fantasy Football League idea. I'd only need a ream of paper and ink for the printer. And a weekly *Irish Independent*.

I charged a pound each to enter and compiled a simple database. I took the weekly results from the *Irish Independent*. I updated all the entries in my database and printed out the weekly league. The £100 first prize went to Barry Lynagh. I made over £400 for the school sports fund.

Previously, I'd organised a hybrid friends' league – eight or ten of us would crowd around in a kitchen or garage and we'd have an auction at the start of the season. Michael Coone was one of these very young neighbours and he went onto win the Premier League Fantasy Football league in 2021.

Would this be a story about educating people on the dangers of concussion? It's not just a risk in rugby, or in American football. It's a risk in all sports; and I'm the evidence of what happens when things go horribly, horribly wrong. 'If in doubt, sit them out,' is the educated position.

People assume I got a big payout for the injury that left me like this. But I didn't see a penny, and nor did my parents, who had to put their lives on hold to look after me. I'd like to think things are different now, but you only have to look at what happened at Euro 2020 or the 2022 World Cup to see that football still has a long way to go when it comes to concussion.

Would this be a story about my efforts to fix myself? Helena is always indulging me in my regular fixes to my splint, my revelatory changes to stretching, exercises, strengthening, physio, orthotics, routine and so on. Even in the car, my position has to be exact. If there's any tiny change to my seat, I feel more pain.

Footwear is especially important: shoes, socks, my splint and the extra insoles in my left shoe. Even wearing loose clothing is important, and a heavy watch on my left wrist as I swing that arm for balance. This combination has been good to me recently. In Australia, I even tipped around Sydney with a heavy book in my left hand to make it easier to walk. People probably thought I was an intellectual or something.

I'm constantly striving for less pain, by changing combinations and configurations of the above. Summer is when it's easiest to change things and try to improve. In the colder, wintry weather, I've learned to just get by. There are a lot more variables to contend with. The icy cold does my body absolutely no good; the wind sends me off balance, as do slippery surfaces.

I visited Sean Boylan and he gave me a rather unorthodox exercise: walking with my left hand on my head! I laughed at this, and forgot about it for a couple of years. Then one morning, running on empty, I remembered his idea and tried it. I felt relief after a few metres, so kept doing it for a few weeks. One stranger said I looked like a rocker from the '80s, holding a ghetto blaster on my shoulder!

The combination of heel raises, podiatry foam toe cushioning, bastardised carbon fibre splint, compression socks, two-toe book stretch twice daily, leg lifts and so on makes it a lot easier to walk the following morning.

One way this shows itself – because Helena works long hours – is that I've become quite the chef. Standing for any length of time is physically taxing, but the kids have to eat. We can't afford to adapt the kitchen just yet, so I've adapted instead.

I've learned that I can't competently carry a pot of boiling potatoes to the sink to strain them. I've dropped the spuds all over the kitchen floor a couple of times. Enter a cheap, IKEA trolley. I can place pots, hot plates and so on onto it and simply push them over to the kitchen table. Nowadays, the kids transport their own dinner plates. Steaming the potatoes is also much safer than boiling them.

Ultimately, as the days have turned into months, and the months into years, I've realised that I need to write this story for me. Not just for the dreams I had – of becoming an Olympic triathlete, shattered by my injury – but for the dreams I still have. I've always wanted to run with the bulls in Pamplona, so that's still on hold. Climbing Machu Picchu will be done as soon as they install a lift.

I can still dream of travelling with my children. I've told them stories of how beautiful Paris, Venice and Australia are, and they constantly hear me talk about Zambia. Maybe one day, I'll bring them to Kalungwishi Street and the garden in number 151 will seem huge again? Maybe Joe will climb my mango tree.

And I can still dream of what science might have in store. This summer, I tried an exoskeleton. It was a magic, if fleeting, experience not to have to worry about falling over, despite my right leg fighting against the robot.

I'm not a doctor, but I do believe that the brain has an inbuilt capacity to heal itself to some extent, just like a broken bone, a bruise, or any other injury. It's a question of finding the method, the key to unlocking this potential. People like Sean Boylan are an inspiration.

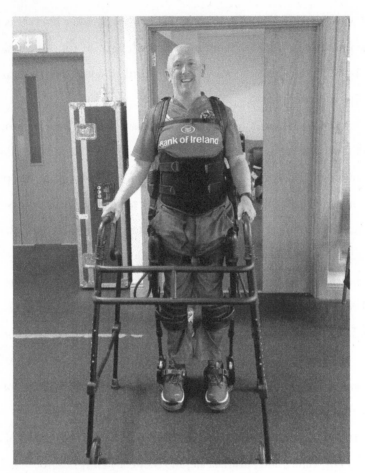

Trying out an amazing mechanical exoskeleton.

Maybe in a hundred years, there'll be a pill that'll fix you up, just like a plaster helps to heal a cut. Who knows? Until then, I must live my life like a non-alcoholic drunk!

Everyone thinks they understand the famous Bill Shankly quote. But actually, if you listen to him speak on what football cost him, the meaning changes entirely.

'Everything I've got I owe to football, and the dedication I put into the game,' he told Granada TV's Shelley Rohde in 1981. 'You only get out of the game what you put into it. And I put everything into it I could, and still do ... I put all my heart and soul into it, to the extent that my family suffered.'

To which the interviewer responded, 'Do you regret that at all?'

'Yeah, I regret it very much. Somebody said that football's a matter of life and death to you; I said, "Listen, it's more important than that".'

After the life I've lived, I know exactly what he meant.

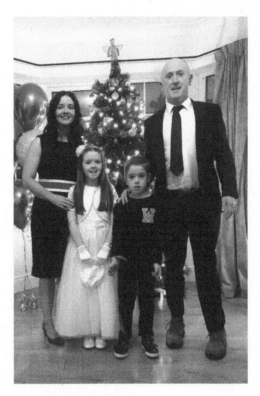

My beautiful family.

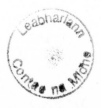

ACKNOWLEDGEMENTS

Firstly I'd love to thank Mam for keeping her diary in '89/'90 and for staying by my bedside every day for three and a half months in Beaumont Hospital.

Dad for instilling an incredible never-say-die attitude and work ethic which I've clung onto. Hopefully my Eileen and Joe will grow up to love me as much as I love you, Dad. You're my hero and a fantastic role model.

My siblings for putting up with me.

To everyone who helped out Mam and Dad back in '89/'90 with lifts to Beaumont Hospital, dinners, prayers, masses said and candles lit. Mam's diary was testament to you all. Thank you.

My grandparents for stepping onto the pitch during this horrible time for everyone.

Michael O'Brien for welcoming me into his publishing house. A true gentleman and I hope I've done him justice here.

Paul Kimmage took a huge punt on interviewing me in 2014. This really put the idea in my head about writing a book.

Shane for getting the ball rolling.

David Finn put a different idea into my head!

Steve ended up being my cosmetic surgeon and getting me over the finish line! He kept me focussed and up when the rejections started coming.

To Liam Hayes who helped more than he knows. Michael Calvin too.

Kevin Mallon gave me the chance to write the St Pat's GAA match reports and more recently showed me the ropes in the National Library, helping me out immensely with all my research. Thank you.

Encouragement came from my ultra fans, Margaret, Richie and Audrey. My cousin Antoinette for indulging me with my phonecalls, countless messages and video calls.

Willie Stewart, Peter Robinson and Emma Russell, thanks for the encouragement and direction.

Seamus O'Grady, the ex-Irish ambassador to Zambia and now Malawi.

Karl Hovelmeier and his PA, Stephen Kasonde. Justyne Kyle McGrath, who advised about our mutual Zambian experiences.

Walter Owens, the loyalist from Belfast who befriended me in Sydney. I learned so much about life from him. Graham, Cathy and Robin in energy marketing.com.au – thanks for giving me such huge responsibility.

Paul Howard and Dave Hannigan guided me, and Ger Siggins was the conduit. Lucinda O'Sullivan for keeping me grounded. Louise Walsh for her encouragement along with Gerry Kelly in LMFM. Barry Geraghty for the nuggets.

Mickey, Billy, Hugh McHugh and Patsy for always being available for a chat and to share their experiences with me.

And Davy Byrne, who always considered me a football man, which meant so much coming from you.

Father Gabriel Flynn and Chris Burke for the regular visits. They kept me in touch with what was going on in school.

To Zak Moran, a few doors away from where we grew up, what a legend. The young man showed such stoicism in what he was facing – carrying on regardless. His sense of humour was similar to my own.

To all my neighbours growing up and today, who've helped me grow into the man I am.

My physios down through the years, from Mary Lynn, Jennifer McGrath and Frank Foley in Navan physio department to Jon Faulkner, Denise Church, Stephen MacGabhann and Lindsay more recently.

To all the staff of Beaumont for putting up with me. Bernie, Liz and Darina, and Carole Walsh who has remained a dear friend. Jenny Robertson, SLT, Cinny Cusack and Patricia Guidon, physios, and Joan Meade, OT. This is my way of thanking you all.

To Eoin O'Brien and Helen Carr, editors supreme.

To all the generous people who wrote testimonials for me, I'm grateful.

To my colleagues, thanks a million for all your help and the slaggings off.

Thanks for all the coffee Stephen, and Johnny for the parking …

To Joe and Lena for welcoming me into their family.

I'm in debt to you all.

To Darragh, best of luck, young man, on your journey.

For Eileen and Joe, thanks for looking after me, I love you both. Keep making myself and Mammy proud …

Finally, to Helena, you're everything, you give me all that I need and more that I want. You speak up for me. You kick me up the arse.

You've always been there for me, so I give you my love with a Bang on the Ear …

Other books from the O'Brien Press

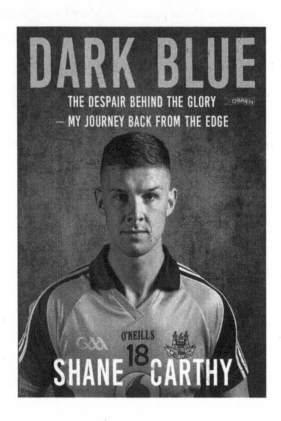

Shane Carthy writes frankly and eloquently about the downward spiral which saw him wake up in St Patrick's Mental Hospital only days after producing a man-of-the-match display in Dublin's 2014 Leinster under-21 final win over Meath. An inspiring story of resiliance and rebuilding.

Short-listed for IBA Sports Book of the Year 2021

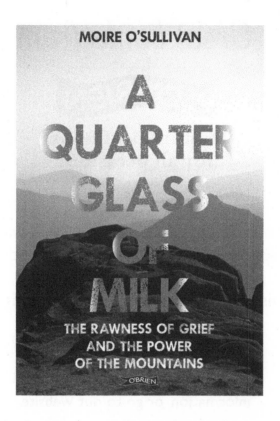

MOIRE O'SULLIVAN

A
QUARTER
GLASS
OF
MILK

THE RAWNESS OF GRIEF
AND THE POWER
OF THE MOUNTAINS

O'BRIEN

When Moire O'Sullivan's husband, Pete, took his own life, she was left with a stark choice: to weep forever over the glass of milk that had just spilt or get on with the quarter that was still remaining. An inspiring story of one woman's path to rebuild her family's life at the hardest of times.

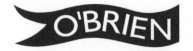
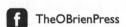 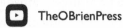
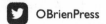 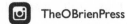